How Not to Die with True High-Dose Vitamin D Therapy

Coimbra's Protocol and the Secrets of Safe High-Dose Vitamin D3 and Vitamin K2 Supplementation

"Learn How Brazilian and Portuguese Doctors Are Reversing Disease While Keeping Their Patients Safe"

TIAGO HENRIQUES

DISCLAIMER

The information presented in this book is not intended to replace the need for a consultation with a qualified medical Doctor and should not be regarded as individual medical advice. The information presented in this book is not and should not be considered an attempt to practice medicine. The author has made every effort to ensure the accuracy of the information contained in this book and that it was accurate and correct at the time of publication. The author does not assume and disclaims any liability to any party for any loss, damage or inconvenience caused by errors or omissions in this book, whether these errors or omissions are the result of an accident, negligence or any other cause. Any references to persons or brands are merely illustrative.

COPYRIGHT NOTICE

Cover Photo Credit © Kevin Gill
https://www.flickr.com/photos/kevinmgill/
License: Creative Commons 2.0
https://creativecommons.org/licenses/by/2.0/deed.pt_BR
Art: Letters and words added to create the cover

ISBN: 9781983353246
Imprint: Independently published

DEDICATION

Anyone who researches vitamin D and vitamin K2 will eventually find, and love, the work of Jeff T. Bowles. It was his first book, detailing his experiments and independent investigations regarding the role of these two vitamins in our organism, which created in me the initial desire to investigate these subjects in more depth.

However, my definitive source of strength and motivation was my mother, Joaquina Henriques. For in her intense struggle against metastasized breast cancer, she created in me the willingness and the desire to search, search for hours, day and night, over many weeks and months. All in our quest against an unrelenting disease.

This book is also dedicated to my beloved wife, Miriam Henriques, who in her fight against ankylosing spondylitis — a debilitating autoimmune disease — has shown similar courage and determination, reaping the benefits of following a high-dose vitamin D therapy in the form of a significant amelioration of her symptoms.

Now, at the end of all these years of research, this book is the result of the inspiration resulting from my investigation of the results achieved by Dr. Cícero Coimbra, neurologist and professor of the School of Medicine of the University of São Paulo, Brazil and his protocol.

All this research has created in me the need to put in writing a detailed explanation of the metabolism of vitamin D and its role in cancer, autoimmunity and many other common diseases, to get this life-saving information, duly referenced with more than 300 footnotes, to as many people as possible.

In memory of Joaquina Henriques, 1949 — 2017

PREFACE

Why high doses?

According to the renowned Portuguese Professor, Dr. Manuel Pinto Coelho: **"Most of the drugs that are taken, try to imitate what high dose 'vitamin' D3 can [do]."**[1]

Furthermore, according to the pioneering work of the renowned Brazilian physician, Dr. Cícero Coimbra, using vitamin D in large doses **stops, and even partially reverses, the damage caused by multiple sclerosis and many other autoimmune diseases in 95% of the cases.**[2]

Recent clinical studies continue to demonstrate the extraordinary benefits, and almost miraculous results, of high-dose vitamin D therapy.[3]

Compare for example the **before** and **after** of high-dose vitamin D therapy in psoriasis[4] and vitiligo.[5, 6] In the study published by Dr. Coimbra with the title *A pilot study assessing the effect of prolonged administration of high daily doses of vitamin D on the clinical course of vitiligo and psoriasis*, photographic evidence is presented demonstrating a tremendous improvement in skin lesions. Copyright laws prevent me from directly including the images here. However, you can check these images for yourself by following the links available in the endnotes.

This is the effect of high dose supplementation in *visible* disease processes.

What about the effect of vitamin D on the diseases we *can't see*?

With vitamin D supplementation, the risk of myocardial infarction lowers by 50% between those subjected to an angiography.[7] The risk of colon cancer can drop up to 80%[8] and the risk of breast cancer up to 83%[9, 10] — imagine! Millions of men and women could still be alive if only they had known about vitamin D in advance. Nevertheless, more than 1 billion people have insufficient vitamin D levels.[11, 12]

Imagine how different things could be for you if you had the knowledge to extract all the benefits of high-dose vitamin D without fearing the adverse effects. People like Dr. Cícero Coimbra created protocols that allow you to do just that.

In this book, we explore in detail the protocols of Dr. Coimbra and other physicians like Dr. Manuel Pinto Coelho. Names mostly unknown to the English-speaking world who are revolutionizing medical treatment protocols.

You will learn everything you need to know, step by step, in a practical guide written in a current and easy to understand language. With simple analogies and easy to follow diagrams you will effortlessly learn all the aspects you must master:

- How vitamin D works.

- The dangers you must avoid and exactly *how* to avoid them.

- The required blood and urine tests and how to interpret your results.

- The key supplements to take along the protocol and how each of these supplements relates to vitamin D.

You will know exactly the *why* behind each recommendation. Think about it. This means there will be no space for analysis-paralysis and that makes all the difference. Moreover, each key statement comes accompanied by references to recent clinical studies from scientifically accredited sources. Nothing of importance is left unexplained or without a reference.

Seeing how everything fits together in a logical manner, you will be ready to share this life-saving information with others, including your doctor.

You will get clear, scientifically validated answers, to each of the key questions:

- How can I be sure *my* body is getting its optimal vitamin D dose?

- How can I be sure I'm *safe* while taking these doses?

- How can I be *sure* high-dose vitamin D therapy actually *works*?

- What is the relationship between vitamin D and vitamin K2?

- How many types of Vitamin K2 there are and how should I supplement them?

All these secrets from the **Portuguese and Brazilian protocols** are finally answered in a simple and direct way in **a single book** in the English language. A book designed to help you understand everything you need to know **from the first day.**

This practical guide is built upon more than **300 references**, providing detailed information on the relationship between vitamin D and vitamin K2 and depression, autism, cancer, osteoporosis, diabetes, autoimmune diseases, fibromyalgia and chronic pain, among many other health problems.

Finally unravel the mysteries of vitamin D and vitamin K2 and **reap the benefits** of high-dose therapy while **protecting yourself from any dangers**.

CONTENTS

Section 1
Mastering The Risks

"Poison is in everything, and no thing is without poison. The dosage makes it either a poison or a remedy."
— *Paracelsus, a pseudonymous for Phillipus Hohenheim, Swiss Alchemist*

"Extreme remedies are very appropriate for extreme diseases"
— *Hippocrates, often referred to as the "Father of Medicine"*

"A scientific truth does not triumph by convincing its opponents and making them see the light, but rather because its opponents eventually die and a new generation grows up that is familiar with it."
— *Max Planck, Scientist, Nobel Prize in Physics*

"Simplicity is the ultimate sophistication."
— *Leonardo da Vinci, renaissance genius*

Section 2
Unraveling The Secrets

> *"Make a habit of two things: to help; or at least to do no harm."*
> — *Hippocrates, often referred to as the "Father of Medicine"*

> *"Wherever the art of medicine is loved, there is also a love of humanity."*
> — *Hippocrates, often referred to as the "Father of Medicine"*

> *"I believe that you can, by taking some simple and inexpensive measures, lead a longer life and extend your years of well-being. My most important recommendation is that you take vitamins every day in optimum amounts to supplement the vitamins that you receive in your food."*
> — *Linus Pauling, Scientist, Winner of the Nobel Prize of Chemistry and the Nobel Prize of Peace*

Section 3
Digging Deeper Into The Benefits

> *"The human brain has 100 billion neurons, each neuron connected to 10 thousand other neurons. Sitting on your shoulders is the most complicated object in the known universe."*
> — *Michio Kaku, Scientist*

"I think that autistic brains tend to be specialized brains. Autistic people tend to be less social. It takes a ton of processor space in the brain to have all the social circuits."
— *Temple Grandin, Professor of Animal Science, Educator and Autism Spokesperson*

"Growth for the sake of growth is the ideology of the cancer cell."
— *Edward Abbey, Author*

"The young physician starts life with 20 drugs for each disease, and the old physician ends life with one drug for 20 diseases."
— *William Osler, Scientist*

"There are risks and costs to action. But they are far less than the long range risks of comfortable inaction."
— *John F. Kennedy, Politician*

The Eight Appendices

INTRODUCTION

What is vitamin D?

The first fact about Vitamin D may catch you by surprise. Vitamin D isn't a vitamin, it's a hormone.[13]

What is the difference?

A vitamin is a substance that our body needs in small amounts and it cannot manufacture.

Imagine our body is like a house in constant remodeling. And remodeling requires new materials replacing the old.

We can compare vitamins with the tiles, bricks and wood being used daily to replace the old materials. Why? Because even though these materials are essential, the builders cannot manufacture them. They can only order them and wait for them to arrive at the construction site.

The same goes for vitamins. Vitamin B12, for example, is essential for the proper functioning of our nervous system. It's found mainly in animal foods like meat. If we stop eating these foods, our bodies will not have access to this substance in sufficient amounts. As such, our nervous system will suffer. How?

When our body starts lacking a vitamin, it begins to warn us with specific signs. The lack of vitamin B12, for example, causes paresthesia — burning sensations, tingling and tremors — especially in the extremities, legs and hands.[14]

What about hormones?

A hormone is a substance that the body uses to communicate with itself. For example, when it detects a danger, our body orders our adrenal glands to produce a hormone called adrenaline. Then, this hormone travels through the blood, affecting each of our cells differently.

Imagine each cell has a book describing its daily tasks.

For example, cells covering our stomach wall are responsible for producing a very important mucus. This mucus creates a protective coating preventing hydrochloric acid from corroding and opening holes in the stomach itself.

We can imagine each of these cells as having a list of detailed instructions describing step by step how to make this vital mucus.

However, adrenaline changes everything. Adrenaline is a hormone, a messenger. As such, it causes the cell to refer to its instruction booklet in an attempt to understand what the body is trying to communicate. What could it be? Let's look at the manual:

Body Manual

Chapter 56: Stomach Cell:

- Daily: Manufacture protective mucus.
- If the body sends adrenaline: STOP manufacturing protective mucus.

Did you notice? This is the striking feature of hormones. They are chemical signals our body sends to **regulate** cellular behavior.

Now imagine your lungs. They have a muscle, the diaphragm, responsible for regulating the rate at which air enters and leaves the lungs. Now imagine these muscle cells, busy with their regular task of inspiring and expiring. Suddenly, adrenaline arrives and off they go, reaching out for the manual, trying to interpret the meaning of the messenger the body has just sent them. The manual is clear:

Body Manual

Chapter 28: Diaphragm Cell:

- Daily: Contract, wait a bit, relax.
- If the body sends adrenaline: Contract and relax quickly!

The same goes for the cells in our cardiac muscle, the heart. As with the diaphragm, adrenaline commands the heart to accelerate.

Adrenaline affects most organs of our body. The diaphragm and the heart explode with activity, the liver releases glucose and cholesterol and this energy and oxygen-rich blood get diverted into the muscles. Conversely, non-essential processes involving the immune system and the production of protective mucus, are put on hold, saving up precious resources.

It's like as if every cell in the human body were a musical instrument and hormones the movements of the conductor. The conductor commands the piano to stop playing while instructing the trombone to initiate its part.

The manual each cell has, containing the detailed instructions on how each cell should operate, is the genetic code. The deoxyribonucleic acid, or DNA, has specific information, the chapters, detailing each cells' functions and how they must adjust their behavior should a hormone arrive in their vicinity.

Calcitriol

Now, just imagine if there was such a thing as a master hormone, a molecule capable of commanding your whole body into a state of wellbeing. At the same time, this hormone would be so vital that if it went missing your whole body would enter into a state of decay. The striking fact is this hormone does exist and is called Calcitriol. *Calcitriol* is the active form of vitamin D3.

When you take a gelatin capsule of vitamin D3, you are ingesting the chemical called cholecalciferol. Then, this chemical undergoes several transformations within the body until it finally becomes calcitriol — as shown later in **diagram 2**.

Due to a mistake when they were discovered, this family of molecules was called vitamins. However, for the sake of understanding, we will continue to use the term "vitamin D" — instead of "hormone D." Just keep in mind, however, that we will be talking about a substance with the properties of a hormone. But, what kind of hormone?

The Super Hormone

Our internal manual, with its chapters, is infinitely complex and, although its genetic sequences are known, we are yet to understand all the complexity of its intricate instructions. However, by the way each cell behaves, depending on whether the body has adequate levels of vitamin D, it seems reasonable to agree with the enthusiasts referring to vitamin D as a super hormone. After all, vitamin D does regulate countless cellular processes in our body.

It's as if the manual of life, DNA, said in all its chapters:

Chapter 56: Cell Stomach:

- Daily: Manufacture protective mucus.
- If the body sends adrenaline: STOP manufacturing protective mucus.
- If the body stops sending adrenaline: Resume the manufacturing of protective mucus.
- **If the body sends Calcitriol: Smile and do your job in the best possible way.**
- **If the body stops sending Calcitriol: Panic and do a poor job.**

Chapter 28: From the Diaphragm Cell:

- Daily: Contract, wait a bit, relax.
- If the body sends adrenaline: Contract and relax quickly!
- If the body stops sending adrenaline: Resume contracting and relaxing at the normal pace.
- **If the body sends Calcitriol: Smile and do your job in the best possible way.**
- **If the body stops sending Calcitriol: Panic and do a poor job.**

At this point, you might be thinking: "Okay, vitamin D is important for my health, I get that. Now, what should I do next?"

First, let's talk about what you should **not** do next. This will be the focus of our first chapter. However, and before we move on, let me share with you an important feature of the book you are reading.

Due to the complexity and importance of the issue at hand, each chapter in this book is accompanied by a summary of the main points entitled "Do you remember?"

This summary aims to make life easier for you, the reader, in three important ways:

1. By helping you to understand and memorize the key points more easily;

2. By helping you to review the main points quickly, without the need to re-read an entire chapter;

3. By providing you with an outline you can use as the basis for a succinct conversation on the topic. This will allow you to share these life-saving concepts with your loved ones or even your doctor in a more organized and streamlined fashion.

The "Do you remember?" summary is divided into questions and answers. To test your understanding simply read the question and keep the answers covered. Then you can review your answers. Don't worry if you didn't remember the answer right away. The purpose wasn't to test you but to exercise your brain. Whether you got it right or wrong, immediately reviewing the correct answers helps you to memorize the main points.

Even if you choose not to test your memory in this way, the "Do you remember?" summary will continue to be useful. This is true because our brain tends to remember more easily the first and last thing we read in each study period.

Moreover, to further facilitate the goals number 2 and 3, at the end of this book you will find an Appendix containing a compilation of all the "Do you remember?" summaries. Be sure to use this Appendix to quickly refresh your memory whenever necessary.

Do you remember?

Questions:

A.   Is vitamin D, a vitamin or a hormone?

B.   In a nutshell, what is a hormone?

C.   A hormone has the same effect in all the cells receiving it? Give an example.

D.   Why is Vitamin D often called the super hormone?

On the next page you will find the answers.

Answers:

A. Vitamin D, in its active form, is a hormone and not a vitamin.

B. A hormone is a molecule the body uses to send messages to its cells.

C. Each cell reacts to each hormone differently, depending on the instructions stored in our genetic code, or DNA.

    For example, adrenaline is a hormone that stimulates the lungs and the heart while concurrently instructing the stomach cells to stop producing protective mucus.

D. Vitamin D is considered a super hormone because it seems to positively affect the entire human body.

How did you go? Don't worry if you couldn't remember some answers, the truth is that now that you have reviewed the main points, this knowledge is more ingrained in your mind, ready to be shared with others who may need it.

Section 1

Mastering
The Risks

Chapter 1

No, Vitamin D Is Not Harmless

"Poison is in everything, and no thing is without poison. The dosage makes it either a poison or a remedy."

— Paracelsus, a pseudonymous for Phillipus Hohenheim, Swiss Alchemist

Recent studies point to a global deficiency in vitamin D involving 1 billion people.[15, 16] Therefore, we now need to conciliate these two facts: (1) Vitamin D is essential and (2) a large part of the human population is deficient in it. As such, it seems reasonable to think the best option for each of us is to go online right now, order a bottle of the highest dose available, and begin to supplement with it.

However, and before doing so, let me tell you about calcium.

Calcium and Vitamin D

Calcium is an essential mineral for life. Our body uses it to correct blood pH, regulate muscular contractions — including our heart's rhythm — and it's the main mineral in our bones.

However, to give our body all the calcium it needs, eating calcium-rich foods may not be enough. Why? Because when calcium reaches the intestine it will only be absorbed in large quantities if there's enough vitamin D available.

That's the problem.

Note the following: Within our neck we have four tiny lumps called the parathyroid glands. Together, they have the function to check how much calcium is in our blood at all times. If the calcium levels drop, the parathyroid sends a message telling the bones to release some of their calcium into the bloodstream. If, however, there happens to be an increase in calcium levels, the parathyroid glands stop sending this message.

To communicate with the bones and the other tissues involved in calcium metabolism, these glands use a hormone called parathyroid hormone or PTH, an abbreviated form used in the rest of this book.

How this happens is a fascinating subject and helps us realize two fundamental aspects:

1. The additional hazards Vitamin D supplementation poses to you if you don't know exactly what you are doing;

2. How you can protect yourself from the dangers associated with Vitamin D and supplement safely — even at high doses.

Your organs and calcium

Again, let us turn our attention to our body's instruction booklet with its fictional chapters. Our goal is to understand the relationship between calcium and vitamin D in a simple manner.

Imagine this manual as having a chapter on the cells of the parathyroid glands and the cells of our bones, kidneys and small intestine. See if you can find out how these cells use the various hormones to communicate. Afterward we will be ready for a brief explanation.

Chapter 8: Parathyroid Cells

- At all times: Check blood calcium levels.
- If there's too much calcium: Manufacture less PTH.
- If there's too little calcium: Manufacture more PTH.

Chapter 10: Bone Cells

- If the body sends a higher amount of PTH: Remove calcium from the bones and drop it into the bloodstream.
- If the body sends fewer PTH: Remove much less calcium from the bones.

Chapter 14: Kidney Cells

- At all times: Filter blood.
- If the body sends a higher amount of PTH: Activate vitamin D and drop it into the bloodstream.

Chapter 21: Small Intestine Cells

- If the body sends Vitamin D: Take up more calcium from food than usual.

What does this teach us about our body's hormones? Let's see.

Calcium Metabolism

As you can see, our body is clever. Being as a vital mineral as calcium is, the body has a whole gland dedicated to verifying its blood levels at all times. And what does the body do when calcium lowers too much?

If it had been me designing the human body, maybe I'd designed it so that the parathyroid hormone, PTH, went straight to our gut. After all, if the goal is just increasing calcium, why warn the kidneys and wait for them to message the intestine?

After all, if calcium has decreased we only need to absorb more of it from any foods being processed at that moment in the intestine. So, I'd put the parathyroid glands and the intestine working directly. But as it turns out, that would be an awful idea! Why?

Well, If I had designed humans, we would die rather quickly. I mean, what if there wasn't enough calcium being ingested daily? What if there was no food in the intestine at a time of need? Calcium is too important for us to take those risks. So, our body has a much smarter way to solve the problem: it uses the bones.

Our bones are a natural calcium reserve. So, if there's insufficient blood calcium, and the heart is at risk of stopping, what is a parathyroid gland to do? It immediately sends a messenger, PTH *(Diagram 1: Point B)*, a hormone, asking bone cells to deliver more of this precious mineral to the blood — *Diagram 1: Point C*. Thus, the body can independently regulate calcium blood levels. For this reason, we don't need to keep ingesting calcium-rich food throughout the day.

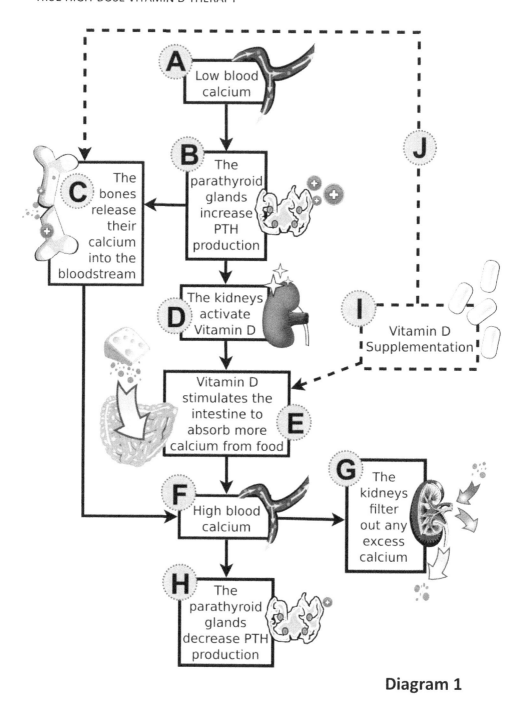

Diagram 1

And what about the bones? Now they have run out of some of their mineral reserves. This isn't good and can even end up leading to a future diagnosis of osteoporosis. We must do something about it. Is it time to ask the intestines to absorb more calcium? No, not yet. Why?

Notice what we know so far about calcium:

- We need exact levels in our blood. Otherwise, our whole body will suffer, especially the heart.

- When there's insufficient calcium in our blood the bones come to the rescue, releasing it into the bloodstream.

Now, notice what we *don't* know yet:

- What about if our calcium levels rise too much?

If this were to happen it would also pose a threat to the heart and the other organs.

Because of this, our body has another important organ involved in calcium metabolism: the kidney. The kidneys filter blood thereby removing any excessive calcium in near real time. So, it makes sense it would be the kidneys the ones responsible for giving the final command to the intestine. And how does a kidney do that? By activating vitamin D — *Diagram 1: Point D.* It's only then, when the cells of the small intestine receive the activated form of vitamin D, that they finally go about absorbing extra calcium from food — *Diagram 1: Point E.*

In a nutshell:

- The **parathyroid** prevents calcium levels from getting too **low**.

When they are down the parathyroid asks for a new

shipment of calcium directly from the warehouse — our bones.

- The **kidneys**, on the other hand, protect us against **high** calcium levels.

  When calcium levels rise, our kidneys filter out any excess. At the same time, it's the kidney the one giving the ultimate call to activate and send vitamin D to the intestines, asking for more calcium.

We are also starting to grasp the intricate relationship between vitamin D and osteoporosis. If there's not enough vitamin D to activate and send to the intestines, the kidneys can't ask for the required amount of calcium our body needs.

Vitamin D and supplementation

Without supplementation it is very difficult to get excessive vitamin D. This has to do with how this molecule is metabolized.

How does this happen?

To answer that question let us learn about 4 different substances.

But there's a problem, three of these substances have strange names and this subject matter can get confusing, quickly. However, I want you to become an expert in vitamin D. I want you to understand vitamin D better than your doctor and to educate him so that he can help you even more. So first let's talk about an analogy that will ensure you will understand everything, even if you have never heard these names before. Are you ready?

Imagine you need to prepare minced beef.

1. First, you take the meat out of the freezer and place it outside, maybe on a table.

2. Then you wait as the ice melts away. But this is only the beginning.

3. Once the ice melts you need to mince the meat, maybe mixing in some healthy spices in the process. The smell is already activating your taste buds, making your mouth water. But it's not ready yet. We are missing a crucial step.

4. The final step is frying the meat on a pan. Now it's ready to be eaten!

Now imagine you happen to be a scientist. Scientists love naming things.[17] So you decide you must give a different name to the meat in each of these steps.

1. "Frozen meat" becomes "7–dehydrocholesterol."

2. "Thawed meat" is now called "vitamin D."

3. "Minced meat with spices" turns into "calcifediol."

4. And finally, "fried meat" changes its name to "calcitriol."

Notice what happened:

First (1) you went for the **7-dehydrocholesterol** in the freezer and place it on the table (2) waiting for the kitchen's ***temperature***, which was much higher than the freezer's inside, to melt the ice. Once the ice melted the thawed meat became known as **vitamin D.** Then (3) you took the vitamin D, ***minced it,*** seasoned it, stirred everything together and got **calcifediol.** As the last step (4) the ***frying pan*** turned the calcifediol into **calcitriol** and finally you got something you could use — or in this case, eat.

Now, notice what your body does:

First (1) your body will get **7-dehydrocholesterol** (our meat) and place it on your skin (2) in the hopes that the *__solar radiation__* (equivalent to our ice melting room temperature) will transform it into **vitamin D.** Then, (3) the body takes the vitamin D and sends it to the *__liver__* (our mincing machine). The liver then converts vitamin D into "minced meat," the **calcifediol**. Finally, (4) that "minced meat" is sent to the *__kidneys__* (our frying pan), where the calcifediol is turned into **calcitriol.** And now your body has finally something it can use — a super hormone prepared to be sent to each one of your cells.[18]

Did you realize how this analogy made everything easier to understand?

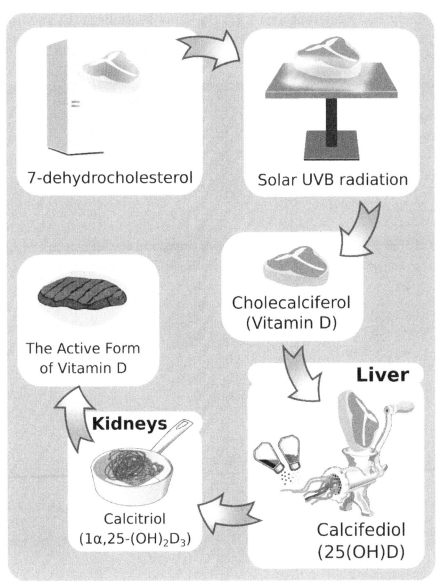

7-dehydrocholesterol

Solar UVB radiation

Cholecalciferol
(Vitamin D)

The Active Form
of Vitamin D

Liver

Kidneys

Calcitriol
$(1\alpha,25\text{-}(OH)_2D_3)$

Calcifediol
(25(OH)D)

Diagram 2[19]

With so many different names for the same substances, it's easy to get confused. This table lists the other common, and not so common, names for each of these substances.

Cholecalciferol — The one you get in most supplements

Also known as:

- Vitamin D;
- Colecalciferol;
- Calciol;
- Vitamin D3.

Calcifediol — The form most commonly measured in your blood

Also known as:

- Calcidiol;
- 25-hydroxycholecalciferol;
- 25-hydroxyvitamin D;
- 25(OH)D.

Calcitriol — The active form of vitamin D

Also known as:

- 1,25-dihydroxycholecalciferol;
- 1alpha,25-dihydroxyvitamin D3;
- 1,25-dihydroxyvitamin D3;
- 1α,25-(OH)2D3;
- 1,25(OH)2D.

7-dehydrocholesterol is just a molecule formed from cholesterol. Solar ultraviolet B radiation (UVB) transforms it into vitamin D.

In this sense, cholesterol is like the animal providing the "meat" our body uses to form other molecules, like 7-dehydrocholesterol.

After the sun has transformed 7-dehydrocholesterol into vitamin D, our body becomes in charge of the remaining transformations, until the extraordinary calcitriol finally comes to life.

This means the total amount of sun we can collect with our skin provides a natural barrier to how much calcitriol our body can manufacture. As much as the liver and the kidneys are eager to turn vitamin D into calcitriol, they always have to wait for the sun to do its part. In that way, you can't get too much vitamin D from the Sun. Why? Because eventually your skin will burn and become unable to use solar radiation to convert 7-dehydrocholesterol into vitamin D.

Any danger lies in supplementation. Why?

Because vitamin D supplements skip one step: our body no longer depends on the sun to turn 7-dehydrocholesterol into vitamin D. On the one hand, this is great news because it means that even if we don't get enough sunlight or even if there's some problem in our body related to the construction of 7-dehydrocholesterol, it will always be possible to increase the level of vitamin D in our blood. On the other hand, it also means that if we are not careful enough we can cause a dangerous increase in calcium in our blood. How?

As we have seen, the amount of calcium entering our blood from the gut is dependent on the vitamin D being turned by the kidneys into calcitriol. If we take too high a dose of vitamin D this will increase the amount of vitamin D that ends up being transformed into calcitriol *(Diagram 1: Point I)* and we will be the ones regulating how much calcium the intestine is commanded to absorb and how much calcium the bones end up releasing into the blood. This latter effect is due to the direct influence vitamin D has on the bones, bypassing PTH.

What is the danger?

By supplementing high amounts of vitamin D, we will be taking for us a role that belongs to the intricate relationship between the kidneys and the parathyroid: calcium metabolism regulation. This means we might be putting ourselves at risk of hypercalcemia.

Hypercalcemia is the name given to the buildup of calcium in the blood. The kidneys are responsible for removing any mineral in excess *(Diagram 1: Point G)*. However, they have a limit as to the amount of blood they can filter per hour. Moreover, when overloaded they may become less precise, discarding other nutrients not in excess like potassium. Also, if the person isn't consuming enough liquids, calcium concentration builds up inside the kidneys and may cause kidney stones.

In any case, what are the symptoms of hypercalcemia?

Excess calcium in the blood causes excessive thirst and urination. It may cause stomach pain, nausea, constipation and even vomiting. Moreover, too high a level of calcium affects brain functioning and can cause symptoms of confusion, mental fatigue and depression.

Another dangerous side effect of excess calcium is related to heart functioning. Given how this mineral is directly involved in heartbeat regulation, high calcium levels may cause palpitations, arrhythmia and even fainting.

If left untreated, severe hypercalcemia can lead to very serious consequences, including death.

How can an excess of vitamin D result in hypercalcemia?

Vitamin D and hypercalcemia, an experimental terrain

If the amount of vitamin D you take is too high, high intestinal calcium absorption will follow. Furthermore, when taken in high doses, vitamin D influences the calcium metabolism of the bones themselves, bypassing the need for PTH stimulation and causing the bones to release more calcium into the blood than they normally would — *Diagram 1: Point J.*

Does this mean you should be afraid of supplementing with high doses of vitamin D?

It depends.

Imagine a man who needs to cross a path through a forest he does not know. He heard about the hidden animal traps and the hazardous terrain conditions. However, he also knows at the end of the path lays something valuable, something that he needs. What's the man to do? He has at least three possibilities:

1. The man should just blindly get on with it, hoping that in the end, everything works out okay.

2. The man shouldn't even try, he should just give up right away.

3. The man should get a map made by someone who has trodden that very path many times before and whose maps have already helped many others to cross that same path safely.

Which one should he choose?

The answer is logical. Likewise, the aim of this book isn't to scare you but to clearly warn you of the existing dangers. If you want to keep safe, you must follow a map prepared by someone who is used to cross the path safely. Fortunately, these people do exist.

Several doctors who are currently using high-dose vitamin D therapy, including Professor Manuel Pinto Coelho, in Portugal and Professor Cícero Coimbra, in Brazil, readily share the measures they routinely take to counteract the side effects of high-dose vitamin D therapy. These measures include concurrent supplementation with vitamin K2 — in the case of Dr. Pinto Coelho — and changes in the diet and lifestyle of the patient — in both cases.

But why are these, and other doctors, venturing through this experimental path? The next chapter will be examining this further.

Do you remember?

Questions:

A. What is the function of the parathyroid glands?

B. What is the role of PTH?

C. Besides the parathyroid glands, which other organ helps with calcium regulation?

D. How does vitamin D influence calcium absorption in the small intestine?

E. What is the effect of a high dose of vitamin D on bone tissue?

F. What are the dangers associated with Vitamin D supplementation?

On the next page you will find the answers.

Answers:

A. The parathyroid glands protect us from low blood levels of calcium by producing more PTH in response to a drop in calcium levels. By contrast, when calcium levels increase they produce less PTH.

B. PTH is a hormone with a double function: it stimulates bone tissues to release more calcium while concurrently stimulating the kidneys to activate more vitamin D.

C. The kidneys.

D. Vitamin D stimulates the intestine to absorb more calcium from   foods.

E. High doses of vitamin D further stimulate bone calcium release.

F. Taking high doses of vitamin D on a continuous basis may cause blood calcium levels to rise too much, causing hypercalcemia to develop.

How did you go? Don't worry if you missed some answers, remember that our goal is ensuring that these concepts are internalized, not getting a good grade on an exam.

Chapter 2

Why Supplement With High Vitamin D Doses?

"Extreme remedies are very appropriate for extreme diseases"

— Hippocrates, often referred to as the "Father of Medicine"

Imagine waking up one day with strange tingling feelings in your feet. In the following weeks, you take a visit to several doctors but to no avail. All of them fail to realize what is wrong with you. Some even suggest it's just some fleeting anxiety — all in your head.

Over time your symptoms say otherwise. Now you go through occasional leg weakness. During those crises, you can hardly walk. Now Doctors are finally giving your symptoms proper attention.

The weeks keep passing by and your clinical status continues to degrade, despite all medical efforts.

A few months pass, and your condition has now worsened to the point where you fear driving your car because you can never know when sudden limb weakness will strike. More medical exams, more medications until, finally, an experienced doctor gives you a diagnosis: multiple sclerosis (MS). Your heart sinks. "Why me?" you keep asking yourself, "What did I do wrong? What could I have done differently?"

Multiple sclerosis is a frightening disease. It can result in paralysis, pain and other serious symptoms. On average, multiple sclerosis can remove 7 years from your life expectancy.[20]

Faced with a diagnosis of multiple sclerosis your options are reduced. They include medication to try to decrease your discomfort and drugs to try to delay the rate at which the disease destroys your nervous system. But ... what if there was another option, a *better* one?

That was the line of reasoning followed by Dr. Cícero Coimbra, Ph.D., Neurologist and Professor at the Faculty of Medicine, University of Sao Paulo, Brazil. Dr. Coimbra's patients are guided in a protocol which includes high doses of vitamin D, vitamin B2, cofactors of vitamin D, like magnesium, and a low calcium diet, rich in liquids.

What are the results?

In an interview, Dr. Coimbra stated 95% of his MS patients go into permanent remission, provided they keep taking an appropriate, person specific, dose of vitamin D. That's right, the disease remains inactive, undetectable by standard testing. The remaining 5% get partial relief from their symptoms.[21]

"Only partial relief" may seem too little, especially when compared with the expectation of belonging to the 95% who report a complete remission. However, when facing the prognosis of a permanent loss of muscle function, the idea that when starting a high-dose vitamin D protocol the worst that can happen is an improvement, this is still exciting, don't you agree?

And what about the damages caused before Dr. Coimbra's protocol? Dr. Coimbra indicates that neurological lesions that are only a few months old disappear completely and the patient returns to a normal life. However, older lesions remain, although inactive — meaning they will not grow and cause further damage.

Given these results, duplicated by other doctors in Brazil and elsewhere, there are at least four questions we need to answer:

1. Where did this idea of using vitamin D in high doses come from? (Answered in this chapter).

2. Why isn't high-dose vitamin D a common medical practice yet? (Answered in the next chapter).

3. How can we take these high doses safely? (Answered in Chapter 5).

4. Could high doses of Vitamin D help with diseases that aren't of an autoimmune nature? (Answered in the third section of this book).

We will now answer the first question.

Where did this idea of using high doses of Vitamin D come from?

Every year, countless experiments are carried out by doctors and scientists around the world. Many of these experiments take place in a petri dish, a flat cylindrical container made of glass or plastic. Thus, even without leaving the laboratory, scientists analyze the behavior of bacteria and human cells and their interactions with many more chemicals. Based on the results they get, scientists weave conclusions about the potential of certain chemicals to cure or mitigate certain health issues.

When one of those theories appears to have sufficient empirical data backing it up, more detailed clinical studies are carried out. These studies may include animals or even humans.

Regardless of whether the results of a clinical study correspond to what the team of scientists was expecting or not, good ethics leads them to publish their results for the benefit of the whole scientific community. Thus, the total available scientific knowledge increases exponentially by the hour. This, however, has led to another problem — which one?

Every single day, endless scientific papers are being published. This makes it really difficult for a doctor to keep track of the results of the latest research being done. In addition, a doctor is a very busy person. He has his personal life, his patients, maybe his own research, his relationship with the hospital or clinic, it's all a lot to manage. Due to this, the doctor learns to trust the system. If a new promising therapy arises, he reasons, it will be communicated to him by the relevant medical authorities. The reality, however, is quite different.

Sometimes it takes several decades for a lifesaving scientific discovery to become common practice. Sometimes it never happens because of the conflict of interests between the pharmaceutical corporations, their financiers and the medical community.

Now, what sometimes happens is that a doctor or a scientist, either because of a personal tragedy or another reason, will begin to do research on his own, digging deeper into the available scientific literature.

For example, in Portugal, one of the vitamin D advocates, using high dose therapy in is medical practice, is Dr. Manuel Pinto Coelho. Taking a closer look at his biography we quickly find out the catalyst behind his personal journey of research. One of his sons suffers from amyotrophic lateral sclerosis (ALS), a very serious disease that tends to kill within a few years. When a person survives longer than expected he is mostly paralyzed, suffering from quadriplegia and maybe even needing the help of an artificial respirator.

It was the love for his son and his commitment to scrutinize the available scientific information that led Dr. Pinto Coelho to come across a whole body of scientific research around vitamin D and other therapies. This acquired knowledge, combined with his own medical expertise, has allowed him to help his son to remain alive and enjoying a relatively stable life, especially when compared to what would be expected of someone with such a serious disease. Television interviews both with Dr. Pinto Coelho[22] and his son, Bernardo Coelho[23] are available in Portuguese in the links provided in the bibliographic references along with a link for an English video from Bernardo's YouTube channel.[24]

In Brazil, Dr. Cícero Coimbra reveals how, at some point in his career, he felt frustrated with the available treatment methods for degenerative diseases. On the one hand, powerful diagnostic equipment allowed him to make a precise diagnosis. On the other hand, little could be done to definitively treat the ailments being diagnosed by this state of the art radiological equipment.

After all, a neurologist has at his disposal machines allowing him to see the brain and the nervous system in detail. High-tech medical equipment like computed tomography and magnetic resonance imaging are a testament to the ingenuity of its designers and the advances in the science of diagnosis. At the same time, after receiving the diagnosis, most — if not all — of the available treatment options involve some sort of symptom control, a kind of assisted degradation.

As we can imagine, it can be disheartening for a neurologist to know that, in most cases, he can only help a patient to worsen slowly.

These strong feelings caused Dr. Coimbra to initiate a search process in the very same databases Dr. Pinto Coelho used.

As he retells, after finishing his training in Jackson Memorial Hospital, Miami, he returned to Sao Paulo, Brazil. He intended to create animal models of neurological diseases, hoping this would enable him to test new methods of diagnosis.

However, from the moment he began researching, he found a wealth of amazing information about the influence of vitamin D on both the immune system and autoimmune disease processes — like multiple sclerosis. He found himself wondering: "Why isn't this information being applied in clinical practice?"

Gradually he and his team grew convinced their patients with autoimmune degenerative neurological diseases could derive tangible benefits from the information they were uncovering. That was information that they had never heard being thought in medical school or at medical gatherings.[25]

After some time digging ever deeper into scientific articles, the evidence kept piling up and the image of vitamin D as a modulator of deviant immune responses become clearer and clearer.

The information that these two doctors have found isn't hidden from anyone. It's readily available in any medical database.

In fact, over the past decades, studies published in the most prestigious publications kept referring to the relationship between a molecule and the most diverse diseases. This molecule is vitamin D. What health professionals like Dr. Coimbra did, was noticing the strong relationship between *high levels* of vitamin D and autoimmune diseases.

Could multiple sclerosis be caused by a vitamin D deficiency? Well, they didn't know. But since its administration is safe — provided the necessary precautions to prevent hypercalcemia are taken — why not test this hypothesis?

In fact, why not? This brings us to the next question: "Why isn't high-dose vitamin D a common medical practice yet?"

However, to obtain a satisfactory answer to this question we need to gain a deeper understanding of the history of medicine and compare it with the current goals of scientific research.

It's worth to note though, that if you are already fully convinced about the therapeutic value of vitamin D and just need clear information on how to supplement high doses safely, you can skip to Chapter 4. Chapter 4 lays the foundation for safe supplementation and chapter 5 builds upon it. However, be sure to look at Chapter 3, because it helps us to understand why it takes so long — and sometimes never happens — for conventional medicine to adopt a new method of treating a disease.

Do you remember?

Questions:

A. Despite the enormous technological advances in diagnostics, what problem remains in the field of neurology?

B. Why are most doctors unaware of the latest clinical findings related to the use of high-dose vitamin D therapy?

C. What were the findings some doctors uncovered as they engaged in more detailed research on the therapeutic value of vitamin D?

D. What's Dr. Coimbra success rate with patients suffering from Multiple Sclerosis?

On the next page you will find the answers.

Answers:

A. Existing official treatment options help relieve symptoms and make the diseases progress more slowly. Yet, most of the times, they don't offer much hope beyond that.

B. Because these studies haven't gained worldwide attention and approval within the medical ecosystem.

C. Some doctors who dug deep into scientific databases found a clear pattern revealing the therapeutic potential of vitamin D in autoimmune disease processes.

D. 95% go into complete remission, 5% report improvement but not complete remission.

Chapter 3

Why Isn't High-Dose Vitamin D Therapy a Common Medical Practice Yet?

"A scientific truth does not triumph by convincing its opponents and making them see the light, but rather because its opponents eventually die and a new generation grows up that is familiar with it."

— Max Planck, Scientist, Nobel Prize in Physics

As voracious as Max Planck's quote might be, it illustrates one of the problems of science. Sometimes it takes many decades until a scientific truth is accepted by the majority. However, it's important for us to understand this same disbelief has protected the medical community from blindly believing each new wrong idea that comes knocking at science's door.

The truth is that a doctor has spent thousands of hours studying, applying and observing the results of his learning journey. He learned that high doses of vitamin D are toxic and that the best thing to do to someone with an autoimmune disease is to relieve his symptoms as much as possible and try to delay the progress of the disease. Therefore, any contrary idea is met with an adequate dose of skepticism.

Skepticism, if not in exaggeration, can be healthy, especially when we consider that throughout his career, a doctor comes across many patients looking for, and trying to apply, different styles of alternative therapies. After too much time witnessing how nothing has worked for them, a doctor's skepticism grows, and he loses some of his initial hope and natural curiosity. Getting him out of his comfort zone and willing to try yet another new alternative approach becomes a difficult task — especially due to the detrimental effect that such an attempt could have on his career and reputation if it were to fail.

And so, we understand the words of Max Planck in a more peaceful light. However, a question remains: If the scientific studies demonstrating the effectiveness of vitamin D in various diseases continue to accumulate — studies which we will analyze more in-depth in section 3 of this book — why hasn't the use of high-dose vitamin D therapy become a common practice yet?

To understand why most scientists and health professionals are not involved, body and soul, in independent research, we must understand some of the history of medicine.

From a historical point of view, medicine has evolved based on case studies.

What is a case study?

In the past, the equivalent of a doctor would administer a substance to a patient and observe the results. Then, this "doctor" would share his results with his peers. On this basis, many scientific discoveries were made. And this makes perfect sense.

Instinctively, this is what we do as well. If my stomach is very upset and I take a tea that makes me feel better and then my friend's stomach is very upset, and he tries out my tea and feels better, it makes sense that a third person, who observed our results, would also feel confident that the same tea, given similar circumstances, would probably help him with his upset stomach.

As human knowledge and technology continued to improve, the focus shifted to finding out exactly what caused the upset stomach and what specific component within the tea, if any, influenced the whole process of recovery. Scientists conducting this kind of research hoped to isolate the active component so that they could study its properties in more detail — perhaps even modifying the molecule to make it more active and safer.

This is the basis of modern medicine:

1. Trying to understand all the chains of events contributing to a given outcome: all the internal processes involved in causing and maintaining a disease.

2. Trying to find the means to influence each of these processes just enough to prevent the result — the disease — from occurring.

From this perspective, we can say that any disease is an emergent process.

What's an emergent process?

Imagine an ant. A single ant behaves like an ant: it looks for food, feeds itself, and tries to find other ants. That's what an ant does. But if enough of them get together, a highly organized colony comes to the life. The colony didn't exist in the ant itself, but was a result that came to life, or emerged, as enough ants continue to interact.

The ant colony represents the disease — the emergent process. It only exists if all the necessary ants can get together and perform their individual roles.

The continued actions of each ant represent the internal processes of the disease. This means if we interrupt enough ants from performing their duties, perhaps by separating them, the colony would disappear, never to be seen again. This is true even if the ants are kept alive but separated. After all, the colony can't exist if there aren't enough ants interacting.

Fire, as an emergent process, illustrates this point well.

Imagine a forest in flames. What can we do?

First, you must understand exactly what are the processes that produce and maintain each of the conditions necessary for fire to occur.

Then we need to find a way, or various ways, to stop enough of these processes.

To emerge and remain active, fire requires three conditions to remain true at all times:[26]

1.   There must be a sufficiently high temperature.

2.   There must be a fuel source.

3.   There must be an oxidizer — like oxygen — to allow the chain of chemical and physical reactions that results in the consumption of the fuel source and in the formation of flames.

With these three processes in mind, what does a firefighter do to gain control over a forest fire?

Depending on the type of material burning, firefighters use different methods that they know will influence one or more of these three conditions. For example, they can use water to lower the temperature or use sand or foam to separate the fuel from the oxidizer - oxygen. Another possibility is clearing the ground ahead, thus removing the fuel source and preventing the fire to spread any further.

Finally, in addition to extinguish the fire, we also want to promote the regenerative processes. And, for a forest to regenerate, it requires the following conditions to be true:

Sufficient trees must have survived. Alternatively, tree replacement processes must be put into practice — like transplanting trees to the burnt forest.

We must make sure the soil has the right mix of minerals and other nutrients.

There must be water available in the correct amounts.

Sunlight must be available.

The logical conclusion is that if a forest is burning, no matter the fire's size, for how long it has been burning, or the amount of people who said there was nothing that could be done: From the moment you take actions that affect the processes that produce and maintain the fire, you acquire control over it.

Why?

Because from the moment you find a way, or ways, of removing any of the three essential fire components, the fire must cease. Moreover, as soon as you find a way to ensure the four necessary conditions for forest regeneration, regeneration happens. There's no other way, it's inevitable.

So how can we deal with any disease? Exploring the inevitability of what we have just described.

No matter the disease we are attempting to heal we need to comprehend:

1. The sequences of events keeping it active.

2. How to stop those sequences of events.

3. How to activate, and maintain activated, the regenerative processes.

Vitamin D and disease as an emergent process

Could high doses of vitamin D help in the treatment of diseases of autoimmune origin or of other kinds?

It depends.

After all, what causes the disease? If vitamin D influences some of these processes, then at least we would expect that vitamin D would have a positive effect on this disease. So why aren't doctors filled with enthusiasm when one of their patients calls their attention to one of these individual studies?

Because many studies don't have a real-life application. How come?

If you search "cancer" and the name of any plant or chemical compound, you will find that there are hundreds, maybe even thousands, of components capable of destroying a cancer cell. Or at least, capable of destroying a cancer cell in a petri dish, in a laboratory, under a microscope and the watchful eye of a scientist.

This scientist, in turn, filled with enthusiasm, tries to duplicate the results in real life. And that's when the problems begin. When a component reveals its potential as an anticancer agent, the next step involves testing it in animals. Unfortunately, many of the chemicals that have worked in a petri dish become a complete failure when introduced into a laboratory animal. Sometimes the scientist doesn't even understand why, but the chemical just won't cure the animal's cancer.

Occasionally, a chemical which has proved promising in the laboratory remains effective in laboratory mice. The expectation of the scientist and his team increases. Maybe he even gets funding for further research. If these later studies maintain the same pattern of good results, human clinical trials will follow.

Many times, this is where the scientists' enthusiasm fades away. A human being is considerably different from a laboratory animal. Scientists quickly get used to this process of having something that works in the lab or in an animal, failing completely in the human.

Because of this, it can be difficult to spark a doctor's interest in the results of a single study.

Imagine this situation: You are a respected doctor. You are aware of the official protocols and you follow them precisely. If one of your patients has an aberrant and unexpected reaction to one of the medications and dies, what happens to you? Even if the patient's family puts you in court under an accusation of medical malpractice, you can defend yourself by demonstrating that you were following the official protocol step by step. That way, if someone wants to raise charges, these charges will have to be directed to the entity who defined and approved the treatment protocol. In any case, by following the established protocols you can protect yourself in court and keep your reputation.

Now imagine this parallel scenario: One of your patients tells you all about this new drug or supplement and requests your help. You listen carefully and decide it's worth the shot. After all, you know all too well there's nothing the regular medication can do for this person. Out of pity, you decide to help. Unfortunately, perhaps due to the disease itself or other circumstances, the patient ends up dying or getting seriously ill. What happens next? Well, let's say the patient's family decides to sue you. How do you defend yourself in court? How do you justify using a treatment that does not have the support of the medical community? Yes, you acted in good faith and with the verbal consent of the patient, but now you find yourself in trouble with your reputation at stake.

This illustration helps us in two ways.

First, it answers the question raised in the title of this chapter and reveals why vitamin D isn't being heavily relied upon by most doctors. The truth is that vitamin D hasn't yet been introduced in the official protocols. This means the experimental protocols with high doses of vitamin D are not part of a university curriculum and nowhere to be found in the medical textbooks. Because of this, if a doctor is taken to court it will be difficult for him to justify his actions.

At the same time, this illustration helps us realize how much the doctors mentioned above, and many others not quoted by name, are confident in using vitamin D. They rely on the efficacy and safety of protocols they developed and borrowed from each other.

Yes, they are risking their reputation, but there's something that hundreds of clinical studies have shown them about vitamin D. There are real, tangible results, that they are getting, and this leads them to continue to put their reputation on the line.

And what about you, the reader, as a mere spectator of this trench warfare?

You also have the responsibility to decide. Yes, there are risks. The biggest risk known was presented right at the beginning of this book. Might there be other unknown risks? Yes, that's possible. The truth, however, is that the latest scientific research, along with the results obtained by the experimental protocols develop by doctors like Dr. Coimbra seem to indicate the risk is well worth it — by a tremendous long shot.

That being said, what is the balanced advice that can be given to you?

Continue reading this book. In the following pages, you will find a detailed description of the current protocols. If you have a good understanding of the Portuguese language, watch the interviews provided above. Check out this book's sources. Read the clinical studies cited in the references of this book. Truth doesn't fear being questioned or investigated, it desires such an investigation. Search for yourself in the forums and groups where people who are doing this type of treatment talk about their results.

Find a doctor willing to support you. For example, someone willing to prescribe the blood tests we will be talking about later in the book. Not all doctors are created equal. Many will be willing to help you. Once you find one, ask your questions and make an informed decision.

The testimonies that populate forums and groups continue to increase by the hour. These testimonies are worth what they are worth, but are nonetheless intriguing to the independent investigator, as you the reader are, at this moment, especially when we compare what these people say in their testimonies with the direction in which the latest scientific studies point.

Having said that, and before turning our attention to these same studies and to what they have to tell us about vitamin D and conditions like autism, depression and cancer, there are two questions that may have been in your mind for a while now:

1. What amount of vitamin D, if any, should I be taking?

2. How can I take higher doses safely?

The answer to these questions will be examined in the following two chapters. Then, we will be ready to talk about specific health issues more in-depth.

Do you remember?

Questions:

A. Why can we say a disease is an emergent process?

B. How can we cure any disease?

C. What is the problem with many promising clinical trials?

D. Why does it take so long for a doctor to start prescribing a treatment that has shown promise in the treatment of humans?

E. Why isn't the use of high doses of vitamin D a common medical practice?

On the next page you will find the answers.

Answers:

A. A disease is an emergent process because it can only continue for as long as all the factors contributing to its development remain present.

B. To cure any disease, we "only" need to discover how to influence enough parts of the processes contributing to its maintenance.

C. The problem with many promising studies is that the results obtained in laboratory tests involving animals don't translate to humans in the same way.

D. A physician is trained to follow pre-established protocols. Doing so protects them from criminal prosecution.

E. The use of high doses of vitamin D isn't a common medical practice because there aren't enough clinical studies to satisfy all the requirements of the medical community, like double-blind, placebo-controlled trials. For these reasons, high-dose vitamin D therapy isn't part of the official medical protocols yet.

Chapter 4

Dispelling the Confusion Between D2, D3, Micrograms And International Units

"Simplicity is the ultimate sophistication."

— Leonardo da Vinci, renaissance genius

Near the end of September 1999, the US space agency NASA lost its 125 million dollars probe, the Mars Climate Orbiter.[27] And why? Due to a conversion error between metric systems. It turns out that the team controlling the probe was using the metric system, but the team responsible for the construction of the probe and for providing the critical acceleration data was using the imperial system of feet, inches and pounds. Unfortunately, neither of them realized that in time, with tragic results for the mission's success.

Similarly, when it comes to vitamin D, it's necessary to pay close attention to two factors. First, one must keep in mind that some older clinical studies used ergocalciferol, vitamin D2, and not cholecalciferol, vitamin D3. It turns out that vitamin D3 (the vitamin we refer to throughout the book) is much more potent than vitamin D2. A study noted a difference of 300% — vitamin D3 being three times more potent than vitamin D2.[28]

The second factor to consider is that there are two ways of measuring vitamin D: (1) micrograms and (2) international units — or IU.

For example, for an adult with, or under, 70 years of age, the recommended dietary allowance (RDA) for vitamin D is 15 micrograms, or 600 IU — 800 IU if you are over 70.[29] However, if you look at a bottle of vitamin D supplements, you may only see a value expressed in International Units, or IU.

Thus, and lest a potential tragedy, it's essential that the reader understands that throughout the book we will always be referring to cholecalciferol — vitamin D3 — using international units as our default measurement unit.

Also, it's mostly in this chapter we will briefly speak of vitamin D2 — ergocalciferol. Therefore, unless there's an explicit indication that we are talking about vitamin D2, the reader can rest assured we will be talking about vitamin D3 — the form being used in most clinical studies. Even so, before taking any supplement containing "Vitamin D" on its label, you need to confirm it's indeed vitamin D3 — cholecalciferol — and not vitamin D2, or ergocalciferol.

What is the difference between Vitamin D2 and Vitamin D3?

Vitamin D2 is a molecule that, after entering our body, can be transformed into vitamin D3. Vitamin D2 is as good as vitamin D3 in terms of potential. However, vitamin D3 full potential is readily available. In contrast, to make use of vitamin D2 the body must work a little to transform it into vitamin D3.[30]

For example, imagine you want to eat a cake. Vitamin D3 is like a cake ready to be eaten. Vitamin D2 is more like a packet with a prepared mixture. This packet has the *potential* to be an excellent cake. However, first you need to join water, stir thoroughly, put the mixture in the microwave and wait a few minutes.

This means there's nothing wrong with vitamin D2. However, why take something whose potential will end up being partially wasted by our body when we can just take vitamin D3?

Unfortunately, some cereals and other products that claim to be fortified with vitamin D, are fortified with vitamin D2. This means you are consuming a less bioavailable form of the vitamin.[31]

In nature, vitamin D2 is naturally found in mushrooms.[32] Just like our skin, when exposed to the solar UVB radiation, mushrooms can produce vitamin D2 in their skin.

When buying a supplement buy one that says "cholecalciferol" or "vitamin D3" and never one that says "ergocalciferol" or "vitamin D2." The only exception would be if it were impossible to get vitamin D3. In that case, it would be preferable to use the D2 form rather than not using anything.

What is the relationship between Micrograms and International Units?

There's no direct relationship between micrograms (mcg) and international units (IU).

For example, 1 IU of vitamin D3 is equivalent to 0.025 mcg of vitamin D3, but one IU of vitamin A is equivalent to 0.3 mcg if it's in the form of retinol or 0.6 mcg if we are talking about beta-carotene.[33]

Therefore, when it's said 1 IU equals 0.025 mcg this only applies if we are talking about vitamin D.

This means the recommended dietary allowance, currently set at 15 mcg, is equivalent to 600 IU of vitamin D3 for an adult, 70-years-old or younger, and 800 IU (20 mcg) for anyone older.

When it comes to high-dose vitamin D therapy, how many International Units are we talking about?

There are reports that in some cases Dr. Coimbra has used up to 200,000 IU daily.[34] That's 5,000 mcg, or 333 times the RDA. Of course, common sense dictates such dosages should never be used without the proper support of a qualified doctor as there's a real danger of hypercalcemia or kidney damage. However, this number, two hundred thousand, gives us a sense of how high a qualified and experienced doctor feels confident in going with vitamin D. Why is this important?

Because, even if in most cases the doses don't reach this number, the fact that such high doses are being safely administered helps us realize the true safety profile of proper vitamin D administration. At the same time, it also helps us understand why most doctors wouldn't agree with this apparent overdose, especially if they didn't have a thorough knowledge of how vitamin D works.

Why such high doses?

Our immune system is a magnificent war machine — until it decides to attack the very body harboring it. Imagine a country where its own army starts fighting against their own fellow citizens. Something similar occurs in the body of someone who has an autoimmune disorder. For no apparent reason, their soldiers go crazy and start attacking the very tissues they were supposed to be protecting.

You probably have heard of various autoimmune diseases like multiple sclerosis, lupus, psoriasis, Hashimoto's thyroiditis or ankylosing spondylitis. All these diseases have in common a misguided immune system. But, depending on the type of tissues that the immune system decides to attack, symptoms will be different.

For example, in some cases, the immune system starts attacking the myelin sheaths. This is the name given to a type of electrical insulation surrounding and protecting the "power lines" of our nervous system. For example, imagine removing the protective rubber that surrounds each of the wires of the electrical installation in your home. Wires would touch each other and could even cause your whole house to catch fire. Something similar occurs in people suffering from multiple sclerosis, causing them to exhibit the typical symptoms: increasingly frequent episodes of paresthesia and the gradual loss of strength until the paralyzation phase finally begins.[35]

In other cases, the immune system decides to attack the joints. Wrists, fingers, shoulders, each vertebra, they all start hurting. This disease is called ankylosing spondylitis. This is a very difficult disease to diagnose. Sometimes, when doctors finally discover what the person has, his spine has already begun to fuse together. The vertebrae literally stick to each other and the person can no longer raise his head or rotate his spine.[36]

These two autoimmune diseases are quite different, but did you notice what they have in common? A deranged immune system. The reason each of the diseases receives a different name is that there are different tissues being attacked. As such, symptoms also change, corresponding to the tissue sustaining the coordinated immune attack. However, the root cause is the same: an immune system that's gone awry.

This is where vitamin D comes into play. Vitamin D is a hormone with immunomodulatory properties. This means vitamin D has the ability to control the immune system.

In simple terms, this means if you keep increasing the dosage of vitamin D you are taking, there will come a point where the dose will be high enough to cause the immune system to normalize and stop attacking its host. When the attack stops, the body will finally be given an opportunity to try and repair the damage inflicted by the white blood cells.

For some people a moderately high dose of vitamin D is sufficient. But for others, higher doses are necessary.

Anyone can grab a vitamin D bottle and swallow a high dose of this hormone, but few people understand how to decide what is the right dose for their specific body and how to ingest this dose safely. The next chapter will explore these topics further.

Do you remember?

Questions:

A. What is the difference between Vitamin D2 and Vitamin D3?

B. 1 IU of vitamin D is equivalent to how many micrograms?

C. 1 Microgram of Vitamin D equals how many IU?

D. In the United States, what is the recommended daily allowance set for vitamin D?

E. What is the commonality between autoimmune diseases and what sets them apart?

F. What is the basic logic behind high–dose vitamin D therapy?

Answers:

A. Vitamin D2 must be further transformed into vitamin D3 before being used by the body. This extra step means the body has more difficulty using vitamin D2 than vitamin D3.

B. 1 IU of vitamin D is equivalent to 0.025 mcg.

C. 1 mcg of vitamin D is equivalent to 40 IU.

D. The recommended daily allowance in the United States is 600 IU (15 mcg) for an adult aged 70 or younger, and 800 IU (20 mcg) for anyone older.

E. All autoimmune diseases are caused by an immune system gone mad. The difference is in the tissue or organ being attacked.

F. In high-dose vitamin D therapy, the dosage is gradually increased until the blood concentration of vitamin D is high enough to exert control over the immune system.

Section 2

Unraveling
The Secrets

Chapter 5

How to Supplement
High Doses of Vitamin D Safely?

"Make a habit of two things:
to help; or at least to do no harm."

— Hippocrates, often referred to
as the "Father of Medicine"

Although the recommended daily intake of vitamin D for most adults is only 600 IU, the general consensus is a daily dose of up to 10,000 IU — 250 micrograms — is safe.[37, 38, 39] Many vitamin D supplements reflect this consensus that higher doses are safe offering 1,000, 2,000, 5,000 and up to 10,000 IU per gel cap.

If daily doses of 10,000 IU were easily toxic we can't imagine these supplements being made freely accessible in most of the world, year after year. Likely, health authorities would have acted to remove them from the market to protect the populations. How can we be so sure about the safety of these vitamin D amounts? Let's see.

According to the Vitamin D Council:

"Exposing your skin for a short time will make all the vitamin D your body can produce in one day. In fact, your body can produce 10,000 to 25,000 IU of vitamin D in just a little under the time it takes for your skin to begin to burn."[40]

Because of this, most people should have healthy vitamin D levels in their blood, don't you agree? So why are so many of us deficient to the point of becoming seriously ill?

For two main reasons: The first reason is most people don't sunbathe the right way. The second reason is that even when they do, there's still a sequence of steps between "sunbathing" and "producing the active form of vitamin D," and many of us have impairments in one or more points of this chain of events. How can we solve these problems?

Sunbathing for vitamin D

Sunbathing is undoubtedly the *natural* method to increase your vitamin D levels. How can we do it safely?

Step Zero

Respect the sun. It's easy to get excited about the idea of doing something as simple as taking a supplement or sunbathing. Consider, however, that these guidelines are for adults without serious skin problems, like skin cancer. People with skin problems need to take extra care and should not follow the advice from steps 3 and 4 of this step sequence, except with medical consent. The sun is a magnificent source of UVB radiation, but it's also a great source of heat in the form of infrared radiation and of UVA radiation. Respect the Sun as you would respect the sea: Just like you wouldn't let your child at sea unattended, you must also take similar precautions in relation with sunbathing.

Step One

Go out tomorrow. As explained above, the production of vitamin D depends on our skin being exposed to ultraviolet B rays (UVB), but glass blocks this UVB radiation. This means if all the sun exposure you have is through the windows of a building or a car, you won't get any benefits.

Step Two

Choose the right time. Just as the amount of solar infrared radiation varies throughout the day, so does the amount of UVB radiation. Infrared radiation is easy to perceive because we feel it in our skin as heat, not so much for UVB. But, as it turns out, the times of higher UVB ray intensity coincide with the times we have always been warned to avoid sun exposure: between 11.00 am and 3.00 pm when there are more heat and light. This means the best time to sunbathe in UVB rich rays is around noon. Of course, remember that we are talking about spending just a few minutes bathing our skin in sunlight and not an excessive amount of time, maybe even to the point of burning our skin.

Step Three

Wear appropriate clothing. UVB rays can't penetrate your clothes. Therefore, wear something that more suitable for sunbathing, while keeping modesty in mind.

Step Four

Make a mental note to skip the sunscreen. Sunscreen protects our skin from the negative effects of solar radiation, while also blocking the positive effects.[41] So what should you do? Remember the goal is to spend just a few minutes under the hot noon sun — an amount of time considered reasonable and safe for most people.

Step Five

Keep yourself hydrated and pay attention to your body. When you expose your skin to the sun, you feel a pleasant warmth. However, after a few minutes, the temperature starts rising. At that time, our body's thermostat switches on. What happens is your body commands the blood vessels on the surface of your skin to expand. Thus, a larger amount of blood will make contact with the surface of our skin thereby moving the heat away from the skin, preventing it from burning right away.

When the skin starts getting pink our body is telling us: "It's time to go find a shade." At this point, choosing to remain in the sun longer may result in a mild sunburn. This risk, and the severity of the burn, increase with the extra time you remain under the sunlight. This is especially true when your skin isn't used to sunbathing. Some people, used to be in the sun, develop a protective coating called melanin — a pigment that darkens the skin while providing protection against sun exposure. Logically, the darker the skin, the longer you'll need to stay in the sun to get your skin pinkish and reap the benefits of sunbathing.

Step Six

Take some precautions if you intend to shower afterward. There's no consensus, but there are some concerns among vitamin D enthusiasts that if you shower immediately after having exposed your skin to the sun you may remove some of the pre-vitamin D newly formed in the epidermis — the outer layer of your skin — especially if you use more than just water to bath. Thus, knowing that about 50% of the pre-vitamin absorption happens within the first 2 hours, it would make sense to wait a few hours before passing water on your skin, to maximize the absorption of pre-vitamin D.[42]

Before you start

Adapt each of these steps to the particularities of your skin, geographical location and climate. If your skin is lighter, making use of UVB radiation will be easier for you. This means you will not need much time to start getting pink. However, darker skins — with more melanin — will be better protected from solar radiation and consequently will require longer periods of sunbathing, perhaps even more than an hour, until an optimal exposure is reached.

According to the *vitamin D council,* you should seek to adjust the time you spend sunbathing to half the time it would take to burn your skin.[43] If your skin burns after 10 minutes, you should expect it to turn pink after 5 minutes in the Sun. Then, you seek a shade. However, if your skin takes two hours to burn you may need an hour of exposure to get the same effect. This approach is especially useful for those with darker skin tones because the darker the skin the harder it will be to notice the slight pink color shift caused by the dilation of the blood vessels in the epidermis.

As for location, consider that the closer to the equator line, the more effective the UVB radiation reaching your skin. Similarly, an elevated location, like a mountain, will provide you with a greater exposure to UVB rays.

Finally, the weather and the seasons also exert a great influence. If it's a cloudy day or a typical winter day, the amount of UVB reaching your skin will be little to nonexistent. By contrast, a summer day, at noon, with clear skies will provide you with the ideal levels of UVB radiation.

As you can see, there are many variables influencing the quality of your sun exposure and the amount of vitamin D you'll produce. Of course, all this provided your body can properly perform **each of the steps** in the sequence of events that culminates with the activation of the super hormone in your kidneys! Thus, it's easy to understand why it's estimated that one billion people are deficient in vitamin D.

Because of all these issues, many turn to supplementation. Still, any amount of sunlight you can get will be beneficial for your health, so it's always beneficial to strive to follow these steps whenever you can.

Supplementation

Vitamin D isn't found in fruits or vegetables. And although a mushroom exposed to UVB radiation provides you with some vitamin D2, food sources of vitamin D3 are all of animal origin — except, of course, for fortified food. Fatty fish like salmon and sardines, as well as red meat and eggs, provide some vitamin D, but nothing like the doses supplementation can provide us.[44]

Therefore, we will now be analyzing how to supplement vitamin D safely. To do this we will be modeling the simple and practical protocols followed by the doctors and independent researchers who have sought to use very high doses of vitamin D — and have managed to do it safely.

Step Zero

How old are you? These tips apply only to adults with good renal function. Children and people with reduced kidney function should not try to follow any of these steps without proper medical supervision. However, **with proper supervision an** **they too may benefit from supplementation with vita**.

In any case, anyone, young or old, sick or healthy benefit from this information.

Step One

Start with 10,000 IU daily. This is the consensus of what a high and perfectly safe daily intake is. It corresponds to the levels we manufacture in our own body after a few minutes of full body sunbathing at summer's noon. So, while you are getting ready to fully apply the next steps, which could take a few days or even weeks, you'll already be reaping some benefits from vitamin D supplementation.

Take note that vitamin D is fat soluble. This means you should eat some fat along with it. This will facilitate absorption of the vitamin in your gut — especially if the supplement you are using doesn't contain any oil along with the vitamin D, such as olive oil or coconut oil.

Step Two

Test your limiting factors: (1) The kidneys and (2) the blood levels of PTH and (3) calcium. The basic tests for a protocol with doses higher than 10,000 IU involve testing the calcium in your urine to access your kidney function and testing your blood levels of PTH, calcium and vitamin D.

After making these tests and confirming that the results are within the normal range your goal will be to continue to supplement with vitamin D in a way that keeps your kidneys and parathyroid glands undamaged and your calcium blood levels within the normal range.

The ThisIsMS.com (this is multiple sclerosis) site lists the following tests used by Dr. Coimbra during the protocol — presented here with some minor modifications:[45]

1. Vitamin B12
2. Calcitriol
3. Calcifediol
4. PTH
5. Calcium (total and ionized)
6. Urea (BUN — Blood Urea Nitrogen)
7. Creatinine
8. Albumin
9. Ferritin
10. Chromium (serum)
11. Phosphate (serum)
12. Ammonia (serum)
13. Complete amino acid profile
14. ALT
15. AST
16. TSH
17. Serum alkaline phosphatase
18. Serum P1NP
19. Serum CTX
20. Calcium in the urine of 24 hours (with total volume)
21. Phosphate in the urine of 24 hours (with total volume)

In addition to the calcium and phosphate blood tests, the following electrolytes could also be added:

22. Ionogram (sodium, potassium, chloride, magnesium and bicarbonate)

I've two reasons for suggesting the inclusion of these common electrolytes:

- First, the intake of water in the amounts required by the Coimbra Protocol, although not dangerous by itself, *may* end up disturbing the electrolyte balance.[46] Just how important is this balance? A disruption in electrolyte levels is very serious and can even cause dementia, coma and death.[47]

- Secondly, the kidneys will be working extra hard to keep your blood free from any excessive calcium. If the kidney starts getting overloaded this may affect its ability to maintain the correct balance of electrolytes, especially in a sick person.[48]

Given how serious an electrolyte imbalance can get, and how relatively simple and inexpensive these extra blood tests are, I say: Let's play it safe and add them to our protocol.

In Appendix D at the end of this book, you will find a comprehensive explanation detailing the objectives of each of these 23 exams. This Appendix was prepared to help you to interpret your lab results and adjust your vitamin D doses accordingly.

Step Three

Understand the relationship between the parathyroid hormone (PTH) and vitamin D. PTH is produced when calcium levels drop. As noted at the beginning of the book, PTH promotes an increase in calcium levels in two ways: By stimulating the bone to release more calcium into the blood and by stimulating the kidneys to activate vitamin D, causing the intestine to absorb more calcium from food. But how does vitamin D affect your parathyroid?

Vitamin D exerts a suppressive effect on PTH production.[49] This means when vitamin D levels are high, PTH levels drop.[50, 51, 52] Herein lies the secret of vitamin D supplementation.

Maybe you have been taking a dose of vitamin D that *you* think is high enough, but if your PTH levels aren't coming down this means you're not taking enough vitamin D. If you aren't influencing the parathyroid, you can't be influencing the immune system.

To illustrate, imagine that a man in Tokyo, Japan is sending money to a family member in New York. He sends them the equivalent of about $1,000 USD every month. Now imagine his amazement when he finds out his family in New York is on the verge of starvation. "How did this happen?" he asks himself, surprised. It's quite simple. Due to corruption, most of the money was "lost" along the way.

At this point the man has four options: (1) Stop sending money to his family, (2) find a safer way to send money, (3) carry on sending the same amount of money, (4) send more and more money in the outrageous expectation that, after all the corrupt men and women get their share of the money, enough would be left for his family in New York.

The same logic applies to vitamin D supplementation. It doesn't matter how much you supplement with, just how much actually ends up being used by your body.

Dr. Coimbra alerts us to this key detail. That's why he pays special attention to the last link in the chain of events: the PTH levels.

It's simple: If your body is absorbing and using the vitamin D your taking, your PTH levels are going to drop. This means that if your PTH levels aren't dropping, your body isn't making proper use of the vitamin D you are taking — whether you are taking 10,000 IU or 100,000 IU every day.

If your PTH isn't coming down, this means your autoimmune symptoms won't go away. After all, just like vitamin D isn't getting to the parathyroid to ask it to lower PTH production, it's also not getting to the cells of your immune system. What are your options, then?

Just like the man in Japan, you have at least four options:

1. Stop supplementing.

2. Find a more effective way to supplement.

3. Carry on taking the same amount of vitamin D.

4. Gradually increase the dose you are taking in the outrageous expectation that, no matter how much vitamin

D ends up being wasted by your body, enough will find its way into the kidneys to be activated.

Of course, the ideal choice, both for us and the man in Japan, would be option 2. However, in our case, there's not a viable and readily available way to directly get our immune system to respond to the vitamin D. Therefore, we are left with three options:

1. Stop supplementing.

2. Carry on taking the same amount of vitamin D.

3. Increase the dose.

If we desire the maximum benefits of vitamin D, we can only go for option number 3.

Returning to our illustration, how could this man be sure he is sending the optimal amount of money? He will have to regularly ask his family.

Similarly, to find out the optimal amount of vitamin D we should be taking daily, we will have to ask the parathyroid if it's already getting enough vitamin D or not.

We communicate with the parathyroid when we test our PTH levels.

In an ideal scenario, low PTH levels would signal us that we are taking the right amount of vitamin D. When we say "low," we mean the lowest value allowed by the reference range. It's only at this point that we will be reaping the greatest benefits of supplementation. Finally, our body will be receiving the vitamin D it needs and this will be reflected in our immune system.

In a NOT so ideal scenario, PTH levels can lower for the *wrong* reasons. For example, if you keep eating foods rich in calcium, like those mentioned in the next step, calcium levels will rise. This, in turn, will cause your PTH levels to drop. But did they drop because you were taking the correct dose of vitamin D? No. So it's vital to avoid all dairy and calcium-fortified foods.

In some cases, PTH can also drop because the parathyroid glands are sick. This is why it's so important to get your blood tested *before* beginning high-dose vitamin D supplementation. In most cases, if your parathyroid gland is sick there'll be a clear pattern in your blood tests. What pattern is this?

Both calcium and PTH levels will be higher than normal. High calcium levels cause PTH production to drop. So, if your calcium is high and your PTH levels haven't come down, this means you have an overactive parathyroid gland. This problem is called hyperparathyroidism and requires prompt medical attention.

Furthermore, some diseases can cause what is called secondary hypoparathyroidism. This means some health problems may cause the parathyroid gland to become underactive, working less and being unable to produce the PTH it should be producing. In such cases, the PTH blood test could be misleading. You would see a low PTH level and conclude it was a sign you were taking the right amount of vitamin D, when in fact PTH would be low due to another disease, like hyperthyroidism. Hyperthyroidism means your thyroid is overactive. An overactive thyroid can suppress PTH production.

Thus, for PTH levels to be a reliable guide, *first* you must make sure you have no illness influencing your PTH levels. This is important if you are unsure of your general health status.

We can compare PTH levels with the needle in a compass. A regular compass is reliable only when there are no magnets around it. The same is true with PTH. Hence the importance of the extra blood tests from step 2, like TSH. TSH levels will help you verify your thyroid health.

Appendix D provides you with the necessary instructions on how to make sure there are no "magnets" near your "needle" and Appendix F will give you further information.

For now, however, keep in mind that our goal is to **get PTH levels down *because* of vitamin D and not just having low PTH levels for the sake of it.**

After making sure your parathyroid gland is healthy, if your PTH levels are dropping it's either because (1) you are taking a therapeutic dose of vitamin D or because (2) your calcium is too high — and acting as a disruptive magnet. The next two steps will help us to remove this magnet called calcium.

More details on how to interpret PTH blood levels can be found in Appendix D at the end of this book.

Step Four

Pay attention to both your diet and lifestyle. To minimize the risks and maximize the benefits of vitamin D supplementation you need to stay on a low calcium diet. This means avoiding milk and dairy products — cheese, yogurt, ice cream and so on. Also, foods fortified with calcium, like vegetable milks or breakfast cereals, need to be taken out of your diet. as an extra layer of safety, bread consumption may also be reduced, especially white flour wheat bread. Appendix C provides you with a calcium-rich foods list and instructions on how to adjust your intake of these foods according to your blood test results.

After all, the more vitamin D you take, the more calcium from food you will be absorbing and the more calcium your bones will be encouraged to release into the blood and, consequently, the more your kidneys will have to work to remove all this excess calcium. As such, blood and urine calcium will be your guide in adjusting your consumption of foods. And as you gradually rise above 10,000 IU of vitamin D you will be taking more and more attention to this aspect.

Other doctors, like the aforementioned Manuel Pinto Coelho, go a step further and recommend a gluten-free and casein-free diet — which invariably reduces calcium intake by cutting out dairy and wheat products.

Drink plenty of water. Dr. Coimbra recommends 2.5 liters (2.64 quarts) of fluids daily, including juices and teas. This extra water is essential to ensure calcium isn't reaching high concentrations in your kidneys, thereby protecting you against the formation of kidney stones.

Limit your alcohol consumption. There's no consensus on the effect of alcohol on vitamin D.[53] There are studies pointing out the negative effect alcohol has on vitamin D and studies mentioning a neutral effect. However, the long-term effect of alcohol on the kidneys[54] and the bones[55] is well established — besides the well-known effect on the liver[56] and other organs, like our brain.[57] For the success of your high-dose vitamin D therapy, you need to do everything in your power to ensure your kidneys and your bones are in the best possible shape. Therefore, be sure to limit your alcohol consumption, especially distilled drinks.

Stress is a big enemy of both vitamin D and the immune system. When you get stressed, stress hormones, as the name suggests, increase in your blood. We've talked before about the effects of adrenaline in our body, but there are other hormones associated with stress, like cortisol. All these hormones change the way our body works, as they prepare us for "fight or flight." One of these effects is all about reducing non-essential processes in our body.

For example, if you need to get away from a bear, your body prioritizes heart and respiratory rate and supplying the muscles with oxygen and energy. In contrast, the goals of producing mucus to protect the stomach lining and maintaining an enhanced immune function, fade into the background. This means that no matter how much vitamin D you take, high-stress levels may prevent your immune system from working optimally.

Regular exercise is an excellent way to manage stress.[58]

In addition to its beneficial effects on stress, deep depression,[59] erectile dysfunction[60, 61] and other degenerative processes,[62] **physical exercise** is essential to stimulate an increase in bone mineral density,[63, 64, 65, 66] thereby offsetting the loss of bone calcium and phosphate induced by high doses of vitamin D. This beneficial effect of exercise on bone mass manifests even in people with low bone density.[67]

How much exercise? If you can move, any physical activity is beneficial. Furthermore, if you have the physical ability and the medical authorization to engage in more strenuous movements, resistance exercises, like weight lifting, are great. In general, aerobic exercise like walking for 30 minutes, may be practiced by most people.

Smoking is another enemy of vitamin D. Tobacco, besides destroying the human body in many other ways, also negatively influences the metabolism of vitamin D.[68, 69]

Some **medications** should be avoided as much as possible. There are essentially two types of medications that cripple the success and safety of the protocol: (1) drugs that disrupt the metabolism of vitamin D (2) and nephrotoxic drugs — toxic to the kidneys.

Unfortunately, anti-inflammatory and analgesic medications, like corticosteroids, usually have side effects related to either the liver or the kidneys (or even both), plus the potential to disrupt your immune system and, consequently, the effectiveness of vitamin D. For this reason, you should immediately report any improvements to your doctor, so that the dosages of any analgesic, anti-inflammatory or immunosuppressive medication may be adjusted.

In addition, you should talk to your doctor about the possibility of replacing your current medication for an alternative medication that spares your kidneys. Appendix F contains a list of common drugs known to be harmful to the kidneys. You can use this list to confirm if any of the drugs you take have the potential to harm your kidneys.

Please note that drugs prescribed by a doctor may be changed only under his supervision. Cortisone and some painkillers, such as opioids, can't simply be stopped or changed without proper medical guidance.

However, if you have medications that your doctor instructed you to take only during flare-ups, you may decide to reduce their consumption for as long as possible. In this case, how could you deal with the flair-up?

There are reports of patients stating how Dr. Coimbra recommends an increase in vitamin D dosing for 3 days to cope with such a crisis. This methodology isn't surprising, because, for example, Dr. Pinto Coelho recommends increasing the dose of vitamin D to 2,000 IU per kilogram (2,000 IU per 2.20 pounds) for 3 days at summer's end to avoid the winter flu.[70]

Finally, Dr. Coimbra alerts to the negative effect that **recurrent infections** have on the protocol's success, notably the urinary tract infections. This is another area where a dietary approach can help. Throughout the Internet, there are reports of people using natural remedies to get rid of recurring urinary tract infections. The methods used often include apple cider vinegar.[71] The vinegar is taken with a glass of warm water. You mix one or two tablespoons and drink this mixture in the morning and as needed through the day.

Other natural methods with some scientific evidence backing them up are also available, including uva-ursi[72] and cranberry juice.[73]

All these solutions can be tried by the reader before opting for antibiotics, due to the detrimental effect that these have on the intestinal flora and consequently on the immune system.[74] Bear in mind though, that a urinary tract infection, when left untreated, can become fatal. Therefore, make use of the natural methods during the first days only. If your infection doesn't respond to them and keeps worsening, you will need specialized medical care.

Some people opt for a preventive approach, taking, for example, the apple cider vinegar mixture daily, in the morning. These people refer several benefits that are outside the scope of this book. Alternatively, especially if the sour taste of vinegar bothers you too much, you may choose to use it for a few days at the first sign of urinary problems — without waiting to see if it's actually a urinary tract infection or not.

Step Five

Take vitamin K2, probiotics and other vitamin D cofactors. For all the reasons already mentioned, and for all the reasons we will be mentioning later, vitamin K2 is the perfect ally of vitamin D. Why? Because it promotes the expression of proteins responsible for removing calcium from where it shouldn't be while stimulating proteins whose job is to take calcium to where it needs to go — the bones and teeth. The recommended dose is of at least 100 micrograms of vitamin K2 per 10,000 IU of vitamin D.

In addition, high doses of vitamin D promote processes within the body that make extensive use of other nutrients, notably magnesium. Therefore, supplement your body with magnesium.

Once again, ThisIsMS.com in its page dedicated to Dr. Coimbra protocol recommends the following:

Four times a day:

- 500 milligrams of DHA (a type of omega 3 fatty acid).
- 5 milligrams of Zinc.
- 120 milligrams of Choline.
- 125-250 milligrams of Magnesium Chloride or Magnesium Glycinate.
- 50 to 100 mg milligrams of Riboflavin — Vitamin B2.

- 1,000 to 5,000 micrograms of Vitamin B12.
- 500 micrograms of Folic Acid.
- 150 micrograms of Chromium Picolinate.
- 50 to 100 micrograms of Selenium.

Once per day, optionally:

- 100 micrograms of CoQ10.

And taking these four times a day gives you a total of:

- 2,000 milligrams of DHA.

- 20 milligrams of Zinc.
- 480 milligrams of Choline.
- 500 to 1,000 milligrams of Magnesium Chloride or Magnesium Glycinate.
- 200 to 400 milligrams of Riboflavin — Vitamin B2.

- 4,000–20,000 micrograms of Vitamin B12.
- 2,000 micrograms of Folic Acid.
- 600 micrograms of Chromium Picolinate.
- 200 to 400 micrograms of Selenium.

Still on vitamin B2, or riboflavin, a study published by Dr. Coimbra and an associate in the *Brazilian Journal of Medical and Biological Research* had the following title: "High doses of riboflavin and the elimination of dietary red meat promote the recovery of some motor functions in Parkinson's disease patients." [75]

In this article, the researchers refer to another study showing that in some populations, notably Florence and London, 10-15% of people have problems with the metabolism of riboflavin.[76] However, even those who don't have this metabolic issue can be deficient in riboflavin. For example, it's estimated that in Europe the riboflavin deficiency levels can reach up to 20%.[77]

Dr. Coimbra and his associate, Dr. Junqueira, solved the problem by administering between 24 and 30 milligrams of riboflavin per day.

Due to the prevalence of deficiencies resulting from a deficient metabolism of vitamin B2 and considering the important relationship between vitamin B2 and vitamin D, vitamin B2 is, along with magnesium, essential during a high-dose vitamin D protocol.

Finally, and being gut health a critical factor in immune system health as it is, adding kefir[78] or other probiotic will be an excellent measure to counterattack antibiotic usage on our intestinal flora.

Step Six

Keep testing your blood and urine every 2 months and adjust your doses accordingly.

If the tests reveal your kidneys are working well and your calcium metabolism is within the reference range, the next step will be to look at your PTH levels:

- If PTH levels are *below* the lowest reference value, you'll need to **reduce** the vitamin D you are taking.

- If PTH levels are *at the lowest value*, but still within the reference range, you'll need to **maintain** the same dose of vitamin D you have been taking.

- If PTH is *within the reference range, but not yet at the lowest value*, it's time to **increase** vitamin D supplementation. This is, by far, the most common scenario. You may increase doses by 10,000 IU or by 20,000 IU, or more, depending on how far away from our goal you are.

Comparing test results with reference ranges is quite linear. Just check your result against the reference range expressed in the column right next to the result, usually on the same row.

A laboratory may use different reference ranges depending on the techniques used when taking the measurements, so you shouldn't directly compare results from labs using different reference ranges. Ideally, you'd find a good lab and continue to use it throughout your therapeutic journey.

Keep a balanced perspective on your therapeutic journey

Now that you understand how to administer high doses of vitamin D safely maybe your excitement has disappeared. Why would such a thing happen? Because you may be feeling paralyzed in the face of so much information. After all, we have just listed many blood and urine tests, as well as many different supplements. Maybe you've never heard about some of them and are questioning yourself about the price tag of each of these many tests and supplements.

Don't let yourself become paralyzed. Even if you are incredibly ill **vitamin D alone** will be responsible for 99% of your results. You'll be getting your B2 just in case you might be one of those 15% requiring an extra B2 dose to properly process vitamin D. Magnesium chloride, which is incredibly effective against a host of health issues — as detailed in Appendix E — and dirt cheap when bought in bulk at any pharmacy. And vitamin K2 because of its synergism with vitamin D. That's it. This is what you need to get better.

All the other supplements might be added at a *later stage* when you're already rolling with the basic protocol. Let Appendix E be your guide. For example, if you happen to be diabetic you'll find chromium picolinate to be a useful addition to any protocol designed to help you with insulin resistance and glucose metabolism. That same goes for heart problems and Coq10, as you'll see.

Start with the basics or you may *never* start.

1. Begin by taking 10,000 IU of vitamin D, 100 micrograms of vitamin K2, 500 milligrams of magnesium chloride and one Vitamin B2 tablet, irrespective of dosage.

2. Take these tests:

    a. Cholecalciferol — also called: 25(OH)D3.
    b. PTH.
    c. Blood calcium (total and ionized).
    d. 24-hour urinary calcium.

3. Drink plenty of water, aiming for the 2.5-liter mark (2.64 quarts).

4. Every other day: try to sunbath until your skin becomes pinkish in tone.

5. Repeat your tests after 2 months and adjust vitamin D, and the corresponding vitamin K2 dose, accordingly.

If at any moment you experience symptoms of hypercalcemia or any other unusual symptoms reduce supplementation to the safe level of 10,000 IU per day. If symptoms persist consult a doctor. Remember that it's unlikely you will be suffering from hypercalcemia if you follow these guidelines. However, each body is unique, and some people may even be hypersensitive to vitamin D, so it's not impossible to suffer a side effect.

Most people will never have a problem, but this book will be read by all kinds of people, so these warnings are required.

Are you a "do it yourself" type of person?

A dosage of 10,000 IU of vitamin D is unlikely to produce the desired therapeutic effect in someone suffering from an autoimmune disease. Why? Because if you have an autoimmune disorder, this is evidence that your body metabolizes vitamin D in a deficient way that ends up wasting a significant amount of this nutrient, as previously explained.

Because of this, physicians comfortable with high-dose vitamin D therapy may recommend starting doses in the order of the 1,000 IU per kilogram of the person's body weight (1,000 IU per 2.20 pounds). This means someone weighing 60 kg (132.27 pounds) could end up taking 60,000 IU daily. In contrast, an overweight person or someone with a lot of muscle mass might need to take more than 100,000 IU per day.

A dose of this magnitude, however, when taken without proper laboratory follow-up could end up causing problems. As stated above, vitamin D effect on calcium metabolism could end up reducing the level of calcium in the bones while increasing its levels in the blood — a process that could lead to hypercalcemia and kidney stone formation.

In addition, given that this type of high-dose therapy is of special of interest to a severely ill person, greater care would be needed to ensure it's done safely.

Due to all these reasons, protocols have been developed that aim to minimize most of these collateral effects, such as Dr. Coimbra's protocol, where all the recommended tests and supplements aim to create the most favorable environment for a safe increase in vitamin D levels - even up to a couple hundred IU.

However, as the reader will have certainly notice, vitamin K2 isn't listed among the many nutrients recommended by Dr. Coimbra. Why? He notes that when administering such a high dose of vitamin D, vitamin K2 becomes irrelevant since it can't possibly be used by the body to metabolize all the calcium being mobilized.

These differing views are common in medicine, especially when we start to get into an experimental ground. The truth is Dr. Coimbra found a method that works and that doesn't include any vitamin K2 intake. Conversely, other doctors involved with high-dose vitamin D are using vitamin K2 in their personal practice. In any case, research linking vitamin K2 to calcium metabolism is far too enormous to ignore, so I maintain my recommendation that you should include vitamin K2 in your personal protocol from the start.

Allow me to demonstrate why.

Bone level calcium loss — a detailed overview

To reduce bone loss, it's necessary for the patient to remain active, walking and exercising, because exercise stimulates bone regeneration. Vitamin K2 doesn't replace the benefits of exercise. However, as we'll explain in greater detail in Chapter 7, vitamin K2 acts in the body as a calcium carrier of sorts.

In summary, although it stimulates calcium absorption, vitamin D by itself, has no power to influence where this calcium ends up being deposited — this is vitamin K2 function. How does vitamin K2 accomplish this?

First, it's important to understand our bones are living structures of immense complexity. In them exists a protein whose function is to attract calcium into bone tissue and teeth. This protein is called osteocalcin.

Comparatively, in our soft tissues, there's another protein, MGP (*matrix gla protein*), whose function is to remove calcium from where it shouldn't be. It just so happens these two proteins are activated by vitamin K2.

This means vitamin K2 stimulates MGP to remove calcium from your arteries. While simultaneously stimulating osteocalcin to take calcium out from the blood back into the bones.[79]

Vitamin K2, however, when in excess may eventually end up reducing circulating calcium levels and, in theory, end up producing hypocalcemia — the opposite of hypercalcemia.

For all this, you must find the correct ratio between vitamin D and vitamin K2.

Jeff T. Bowles, an independent researcher who published a book detailing his personal experiences with high doses of vitamin D, recommends a vitamin K2 supplement that contains 1,000 mcg of vitamin K2 MK-4 and 200 micrograms of vitamin MK-7 — more about the difference between MK-4 and MK-7 in chapter 7. He recommends taking one of these gel capsules per 10,000 IU of vitamin D.[80]

This means someone weighing 60 kg (132.27 pounds), would end up taking 60,000 IU of vitamin D and 7,200 mcg of vitamin K2 — 6,000 in MK-4 form and 1,200 mcg in MK-7 form.

Dr. Manuel Pinto Coelho is much more conservative in this respect, recommending 100 micrograms of vitamin K2 per 10,000 IU of vitamin D — without specifying if MK-4 or MK-7.[81] He also prescribes Herbensurina[82, 83] tea to promote calcium excretion and reduce kidney stone formation risks. It's also worth mentioning, especially if you are still concerned about the possibility of using vitamin D doses above 10,000 IU, that Dr. Pinto Coelho states he hasn't seen any case of vitamin D induced hypercalcemia.[84] This illustrates how well our body is at regulating blood calcium levels, especially under proper medical supervision that includes vitamin K2.

In fact, even if the amount of calcium being mobilized by high-dose vitamin D is far superior to vitamin K2 ability to handle it all, no one can deny the beneficial effect of supplementing with a molecule that promotes calcium transportation to the right place. Moreover, as we shall see in Chapter 7, this is just *one* of the many reasons to include vitamin K2 supplements in our own protocol.

It wouldn't be too farfetched to imagine that high-dose concurrent supplementation with vitamin K2 could act as a buffer against that day you fail to drink enough water or inadvertently end up consuming a calcium-rich food.

Conclusion

Now that we understand how to safely supplement with high doses of vitamin D, it's time to understand at a much deeper level why this "vitamin" is so vital to us. This extra knowledge is so important because it can act as a motivating force during our healing journey, even if the results we desire take longer than expected to appear. Moreover, understanding *why* will help you firm your hope in solid ground and provide you with an exact knowledge you can share with others.

Important warning

Because of the close relationship between vitamin K2 and vitamin K1, **if you are taking anticoagulants you absolutely need to consult your doctor before taking vitamin K2.** Also, if you are taking the pill[85] or any other drug with an associated risk of clot creation you should consult with a doctor before supplementing with either vitamin K1 or K2. This extra layer of safety will assure you the best of results in the safest manner.

Do you remember?

Questions:

A. What is the safe vitamin D upper limit according to most vitamin D experts?

B. What are the 6 steps to sunbathe safely and effectively?

C. What are the 6 steps to supplement vitamin D safely and effectively?

D. What is the vitamin D starting dose used in experimental protocols?

E. What is the variation in the dose of vitamin K2 used in experimental protocols?

Answers:

A. The general accepted vitamin D upper limit among vitamin D experts is 10,000 IU — 250 micrograms.

B. The six steps to sunbathe safely and effectively are: (1) Going out into the sun. Afterall, glass blocks UVB. (2) Choosing the best time interval, between 11:00 am and 3:00 pm. (3) Don't cover your entire body with clothes. Clothes block UVB radiation just like glass does. (4) Don't wear sunscreen. (5) Sunbath for just long enough for your skin to start turning pink. As a rule of thumb this means sunbathing for half the time it would take sunlight to burn your skin. (6) Take a bath only a few hours after sun exposure.

C. The six steps to supplement vitamin D safely and effectively are: (1) Start with 10,000 IU per day. (2) Test your kidneys by measuring 24-hour urinary calcium and checking your blood levels of calcium, PTH and vitamin D with the 25(OH)D or 25-hydroxycholecalciferol test. (3) Understand the goal isn't just to increase vitamin D blood levels. Your focus is lowering blood PTH levels to the minimum allowed by the reference range. (4) Reduce consumption of calcium, increase the consumption of water and seek to lead a physically active life without too much stress. (5) Supplement at least with vitamin K2, vitamin B2 and magnesium chloride. (6) Repeat the blood tests periodically and adjust your vitamin D and vitamin K2 doses accordingly.

D. The base dosage used on experimental protocols is 1,000 IU of vitamin D per kilogram of body weight (1,000 IU per 2.20 pounds). This dosing is then either increased or decreased according to lab results.

E. The common dose of vitamin K2 used is of 100 mcg per 10,000 IU of vitamin D. Although in some cases it can get much higher. The independent researcher Jeff T. Bowles recommends 200 mcg of vitamin K2 MK-7 taken together with 1,000 mcg of vitamin K2 MK-4 per 10,000 IU of vitamin D.

Chapter 6

Vitamin D and the Immune System — the science behind high-dose therapy

"Wherever the art of medicine is loved, there is also a love of humanity."

— Hippocrates, often referred to as the "Father of Medicine"

I magine you are driving your car on the highway. Suddenly the driving wheel stops responding. You try to brake but the car does not react. What would you do?

Something similar happens in autoimmune diseases. It's estimated that at any given moment we will have between 4,000 and 10,000 white blood cells per microliter of blood — an average of 7,000.[86] The average human has about 5 liters of blood in his body[87] — 5,000,000 microliters. This means we have, on average, 35 billion white blood cells within us. This means within each of us there's an army of 35 billion soldiers. That's more than 4 times the Earth's population.

Now imagine this army of galactic proportions is under your command. But there's a problem. All your communication systems are from the First World War era. Let this idea sink in for a moment.

Well, "this is like driving a car with no brakes and no steering wheel!" you might think. And you'd be right. Now, **this is the same impossible challenge that your body is facing when it tries to coordinate tens of billions of white blood cells without enough vitamin D available.**

To make matters worse, many people have a genetic resistance to vitamin D. This means they have one or more flaws along the chain of events culminating in the use of vitamin D to control the immune system.

This chain of events begins when your body makes 7-dehydrocholesterol from cholesterol and depends on a harmonious dance between UVB rays and our skin, liver, kidneys, parathyroid glands and numerous enzymes and chemical reactions.

In addition, many drugs interfere with either the absorption or the metabolism of vitamin D, effectively jamming the communication lines with the immune system.

Adding to this, we learned to stay out of the sun around noon, the time when UVB radiation is at its strongest intensity.

We have a multifactorial recipe for disaster. This disaster it's called an autoimmune condition.

This is the inescapable truth: Without proper communication lines a man can't command his army, no matter what his military credentials are. Similarly, without vitamin D a body can't exercise proper control over any immune system — why?

What is the role of vitamin D in all this?

If we recall, vitamin D is a substance that our body can transform into a super hormone — calcitriol: a messenger that modifies the work of our cells. When activated, vitamin D enters the blood, affecting much more than calcium metabolism. In fact, it affects the expression of many genes in our genome, between 3 to 10% of our genes — depending on the source consulted.[88] Many of our immune cells have vitamin D receptors, meaning that they have "secret" functions, pages and pages of instructions in their manuals that they only read and execute when the activated vitamin D comes into contact with them.[89, 90]

Another key point is that the immune system has a type of cell called regulatory T cell, responsible for suppressing the immune system. If the immune system is like a car, then the regulatory T cell is the brake. And as was expected, it's vitamin D that stimulates the production of this lymphocyte.[91] Without a braking mechanism, how you will stop the immune system from performing a misguided attack?

Moreover, some types of immune cells use vitamin D to communicate with each other by mimicking the kidneys and converting vitamin D into calcitriol.[92]

For all this, it's no wonder that this same substance, vitamin D, can positively influence so many types of diseases.

After all, from the moment we managed to get control over an army of galactic proportions it becomes obvious why cancer will have a much harder time developing. As soon as the first cancer cell arises it will face our specialized troops, and, with the help of vitamin D, the immune system will be much more able to perform its duty of protecting us from harm.

But there's another aspect connecting the immune system, and therefore vitamin D, with countless diseases. By understanding this aspect you'll understand even better why vitamin D exerts such a beneficial and positive effect on the human body. This aspect is inflammation.

What is inflammation?

Inflammation is the at the root of many modern diseases, but what is inflammation?

One of the special abilities of our immune cells involves the production of chemicals that help us survive.

When the immune system detects an intruder, like a bacterium, it works together to produce specific chemicals designed to destroy the invader. In addition, several types of white blood cells work together to send messages — through hormones — to all the other members of the army, informing them of what was detected and how it can be destroyed.

In addition, white blood cells release chemicals that increase blood and fluid flow to the tissue sustaining the attack. This causes a swelling of the area and an increase in temperature. These defensive processes are vital because they will kill some of the invading pathogens while increasing the body's ability to, among other things, send more white blood cells to the area faster.

So, when we say an area of the body is inflamed, we are literally saying that our white blood cells began to release chemicals (1) to destroy intruders and to (2) stimulate an increase in the amount of blood and fluids serving the area.

These protective actions transform our tissues from into a real battlefield. This has some nasty side effects. One of them is tissue degeneration. This degeneration occurs as follows:

1. As the immune system continues to attack the intruder, the destructive chemicals being produced will also damage the surrounding tissues. Imagine the police is having a long exchange of gunshots with a group of heavily armed criminals — in a museum. What would happen to the

museum? As we may imagine, it would have to be closed for reparation for a long time.

2. Also, as the body continues to respond to the request to divert blood and fluid to the area, all that extra pressure will cause tissue irritation and swelling. This ends up promoting a faster degradation of those cellular structures.

For these reasons, and in normal situations, the inflammatory response is activated only when it is really necessary and for a limited period.

This means whenever our body allows the inflammatory response to be active longer than required needless destruction of our tissues occurs. This causes all sorts of symptoms, depending on the organ system sustaining the inflammatory attack.

Autoimmunity and inflammation

If the immune system is malfunctioning, it can detect that a part of our body that is working fine, must be destroyed. Since we are talking about a part of our body that is **fine,** it will never turn into something else. Unfortunately, this means our immune system will never stop attacking it until the targeted tissue is destroyed. And how does the immune system attacks? By activating inflammatory processes. Or, in other words, by firing harmful chemicals at the unsuspecting tissues and by influencing the body to send blood and fluids to the area — further increasing the fragility of the tissues, making them even more vulnerable to the chemical attack. Our joints are one of the most sensitive tissues we have, hence they are frequently affected by various types of autoimmune disorders.

Immunosuppression and the inflammatory response

If someone has an autoimmune disease, at some point he will be asked to start immunosuppressant medication. These are drugs that attempt to prevent the immune system from attacking the body.

How do they work? To understand this, we must dig deeper into the inner workings of the inflammatory response.

Attacking its own body is a basic function of a healthy immune system. For example, whenever a cell divides incorrectly, the immune system has a vital role in preventing this cell from further divisions. If it fails to do so, the person will develop a focus of cancer. This means that all the time, our immune system makes hundreds, or perhaps thousands, of attacks aimed at our own body — attacks that keep us healthy.

Also, inflammation, in itself, is something natural, as is a fever. When it detects an intruder, our organism raises its temperature. This serves several purposes, like allowing white blood cells to move faster. In addition, high temperature, by itself, can kill many harmful microbes. Similarly, inflammation — the production of destructive chemicals and the increase in fluid and blood circulation to the affected area — allows for a greater ability to attack intruders and in some cases, like a skin cut, it can even help with tissue regeneration.

This means using drugs designed to prevent the immune system from functioning isn't the ideal way to solve the problem of autoimmunity. Still, using these drugs is preferable compared with doing nothing and letting autoimmunity run rough until you are finally paralyzed or even dead. Although in most cases these drugs don't prevent this tragic outcome, they have the potential to push it away for a while.

How do immunosuppressant drugs work?

An attack of the immune system, either directed against its own body or at an intruder, is the final result of a chain of events. This isn't "detect and decide to attack" in a single step. This is good news because it means there are many intermediate steps in between detection of a problem and the actual attack. All these intermediary steps represent an opportunity to intervene and stop an incorrect inflammatory response.

The attack, the latest action in this chain of events, occurs with the production of cytokines. Cytokines are one of the chemicals capable of destroying whatever they contact. They are produced by neutrophils and other white blood cells. Neutrophils are "blind." They don't distinguish bad from good, friend from foe. When they are activated they produce cytokines. Who is activating them? Other immune system cells, which in turn, are just reacting to the evaluations and decisions made by previous immune cells, all of them taking part in a complex exchange of chemical messages.

We can compare a cytokine with a thermonuclear missile. To launch a missile, a series of steps are needed, like entering secret codes and rotating safety keys. However, when the final order comes, there's nothing that the man behind the trigger can do. He is like the neutrophil, he just follows orders. However, all this bureaucracy preceding a missile launch exists due to the fearsome destructive power that a nuclear weapon has.

Similarly, our body has several safety mechanisms in place to prevent neutrophils from damaging the body more than necessary. First, there's the sequence of events that must be coordinated between the various immune cells — from the detection of an intruder to the production of the inflammatory chemicals. Beyond that, there's also an additional security measure: contrary to other cells, with a longer lifespan, neutrophils only live little more than five days.[93]

This means that in normal situations, even an intense inflammatory response triggered by mistake would never last more than a few days. In addition, there are cells that produce chemicals that suppress inflammation, like the already mentioned regulatory T cell.[94] All this ensures the destructive power of the immune system remains under tight control.

In that case, how can an inflammatory response last for **decades**?

As we can see, such as tremendous failure in modulating the inflammatory response must be attributed to an equal phenomenal sequence of mistakes.

Therefore, we realize that an autoimmune disease must be the result of a multitude of failures in immune system modulation. Drugs try to solve the problem creating *even more* flaws. Their goal is disabling the immune system.

Certain immunosuppressive drugs, for example, suppress the free flow of TNF — Tumor Necrosis Factor — itself a cytokine, and one of the many chemicals the immune system cells use to communicate.[95]

So, the attack on our joints is reduced, but so is the attack against existing cancer cells, invading bacteria and multiplying viruses.

The therapy with vitamin D, on the other hand, is the result of an entirely different way of thinking. When using vitamin D, instead of asking, "How can I force the immune system to stop the inflammatory response?" the health professional is actually wondering: "How can I reactivate the security mechanisms ensuring the inflammatory response is activated only when needed?" This paradigm shift, rather than further reduce the communication capacity of the entire immune system, aims to give it what it needs to function optimally — vitamin D.

Thus, with this knowledge in mind, we now return to the mental exercise we carried out in chapter 3.

What would you do?

Imagine this situation: You are a respected doctor. You are aware of the official protocols and you follow them precisely. But now a man with multiple sclerosis stands in front of you. It tells you all about his suffering, how his legs are losing function and how much it all hurts day and night. You look carefully at the MRI and realize that in a few more months this man will be paralyzed.

He shows you the prescription drugs he has been taking. It's the common medication, so you understand the disease may take a little longer to develop, but the prognosis is still poor. Two years max and this man will be confined to a wheelchair – for life.

What will you do?

"Well I can't do anything," you think. Then you remember: "I know how to administer high doses of vitamin D safely. I know what the medical literature says about their immunomodulatory properties. I know cases of people who are following a high-dose protocol and went into remission. I know I can change the fate of this man."

What will you do?

However great your fear that something unexpected can go wrong, you feel a moral obligation to help this poor man. It's this same desire to help his fellow man that moves a physician like Dr. Coimbra into action.

Conclusion

The research and the practical applications surrounding vitamin D, although experimental, are certainly impressive. The benefits of supplementation, when under the supervision of an informed health professional give much hope to those who are suffering. But what about vitamin K2?

As we had the opportunity to observe in Chapter 5, vitamin K2 is directly related to calcium metabolism and some doctors and independent researchers are actively recommending it as an essential part of a high-dose vitamin D protocol. In the next chapter we analyze more thoroughly what vitamin K2 is and how you can benefit from it.

Do you remember?

Questions:

A.   What is inflammation?

B.   What are the positive aspects of the inflammatory response?

C.   What are the negative aspects of the inflammatory response?

D.   How do immunosuppressants drugs work?

E.   What is the name of the white blood cell responsible for stopping the inflammatory response?

F.   How does vitamin D differ from immunosuppressants in its mechanism of action?

Answers:

A. When it detects an intruder or a cell of the body that needs to be destroyed — like a cancer cell — the immune system produces chemicals aimed at destroying the enemy while at the same time stimulating the body to send more blood and fluids to the area.

B. The extra blood and fluids reaching the affected area carry with them nutrients and platelets, which promotes healing, and more immune cells. In addition, extra fluids serve as a blockade against the propagation of intruders.

C. Inflammatory cytokines and other chemicals released during an extended inflammatory response cause irritation and damage to the surrounding healthy tissues.

D. Immunosuppressant drugs attempt to interrupt the chain of events that leads to the activation of a full-blown inflammatory response.

E. The white blood cell responsible for stopping the inflammatory response is called regulatory T cell.

F. Vitamin D enhances the communication within the immune system and promotes the production of regulatory T cells.

Chapter 7

Vitamin K2 — Making Friends With the Unknown Healer

"I believe that you can, by taking some simple and inexpensive measures, lead a longer life and extend your years of well-being. My most important recommendation is that you take vitamins every day in optimum amounts to supplement the vitamins that you receive in your food."

— Linus Pauling, Scientist, Winner of the Nobel Prize of Chemistry and the Nobel Prize of Peace

Worldwide, heart disease is the deadliest disease.[96] It develops silently and often the first symptom is a heart attack. For this reason, doctors are always looking for ways to evaluate who is at risk before this first, and often last, sign of heart disease appears.

What was discovered is that the buildup of calcium in the arteries feeding the heart is one of the major risk factors.[97] This means the more calcium you have accumulated in your coronary arteries the greater your chances of suffering a heart attack.

With this in mind, wouldn't it be great if there was a way to remove this calcium from where it shouldn't be? Even better: What if, in addition to removing calcium from where it shouldn't be, we could make it useful again? Maybe by moving it to where it's *needed*, like our bones and teeth.

A substance of this sort would be extraordinary. Fortunately, this substance exists. Unfortunately, it's virtually unknown. It's called vitamin K2.[98]

If you have never heard your heart doctor mentioning vitamin K2 that's not surprising. For many decades it was considered that vitamin K2 had no relevant function. This helps us to realize why the public is still unaware of vitamin K2.[99]

Let's undo this unfortunate problem.

The origins of the "K"

Vitamin K was first discovered in 1929 by a Danish scientist named Henrik Dam. He noted this new molecule was directly related to blood clotting, so he called it *koagulationsvitamin* using the words "coagulation" and "vitamin."

Today, this molecule, essential in the process of blood clotting, is called vitamin K1. This "1" is added to distinguish it from a closely related molecule, the aforementioned vitamin K2. Now, what could be the relationship between a molecule that aids in blood clotting, vitamin K1, and a molecule that helps the body in moving calcium from soft tissues into bone? Let's find out.

The relationship between vitamin K1, vitamin K2 and calcium

When we wound our skin, our body sends platelets to seal the cut. This process is called coagulation and serves two purposes. First, it prevents the loss of blood and other fluids through the opening. Secondly, the barrier created by the platelet cluster acts as a perfect restriction against the entry of bacteria and other opportunistic invaders.

But, how does calcium relate to this clotting process?

If you have had the opportunity to so some bricolage, you probably used silicone glue or some type of plaster preparation. You probably also noticed that, while the product dried up, it left an unpleasant smell in the air.

That smell you felt is caused by the chemicals acting as diluents. These ensure the product will stay soft for as long as it remains within its original packaging. When the product leaves the container, the diluent begins to evaporate. Simultaneously, the product reacts with the oxygen in the air and all that creates several more chemical reactions that cause the product to gradually harden.

Something similar happens with our blood.

In its natural state blood is very fluid. Although it contains many white and red blood cells, platelets and a multitude of nutrients and hormones — in addition to many other molecules — it remains quite diluted. This feature is great because it allows blood to freely flow throughout all kinds of blood vessels, feeding our cells.

However, if you leave blood in contact with air, what happens? It hardens, or clots. What happened to blood is like how the sealants and plasters of industrial origin work. The oxygen in the air reacts with a protein that exists in platelets called scramblase. Upon activation, scramblase initiates its job. Scramblase has the responsibility of transporting negatively charged phospholipids all the way from the inside of platelets to the outside. Outside, these phospholipids create a platform where various chemicals can now react with each other to activate blood clotting.[100]

The body machinery is fascinating.

We can imagine the platelet as a woodworking vault, with a high-security door. To get inside, a special identification is required. Only scramblase has this identification. But scramblase is like a sleeping doorkeeper. So, if you want to use the wooden table inside the platelet's vault, you need to wake up the doorkeeper and ask him to go get the table inside.

The table represents the negatively charged phospholipids and the platform they form when they get outside the platelet. Then scramblase — the doorkeeper — brings out this table, piece by piece, and assembles it. At that moment, on the phospholipid platform — the table — many chemical reactions begin to take place, culminating with the clotting of a small portion of blood.

It all started with waking up the doorkeeper. Now, can you guess what is the substance that wakes him up? That's right, it's calcium. In normal situations the calcium concentration inside the platelet is very low, but when there's a need to activate coagulation our body finds a way to send calcium into the platelet.

In short, calcium is used to activate scramblase and scramblase is used to load and assemble "the table of phospholipids" on the outer wall of the platelet. Now we only need to build the fibrils, which are like a mesh of nearly indestructible threads involving platelets and contributing to the creation of the clot.

But building the fibrils on top of the phospholipids table is still an incredibly complex process. Calcium plays a key role here too, as it is a dication. This means he has two arms. With an arm, calcium grabs the phospholipid table and with the other arm, it grasps for a chemical. Thus, many calcium dications will act as a magnet, forcing all the needed chemicals to stay in place, at the table, for the time required for the reactions to occur.

These chemicals react in what is called the coagulation cascade and at the end of this process, fibrils come to life. The fibrils cause the blood plasma to turn into a kind of gel. Blood cells and plasma are then entangled in the network of fibrils, forming a clot.

What about vitamin K1?

Vitamin K1 was always present. Why can we say that? Because several of those substances that calcium picked up and brought to the "table" of phospholipids were vitamin K1 dependent. What does this mean? It means the molecule called vitamin K1 has a format that fits these clotting factors and modifies them to allow them to be used in the chemical reactions required to build up the fibrils. Without vitamin K1 calcium wouldn't be able to interact with the clotting factors. It's like vitamin K1 is a master key, and each of the coagulation factors needed that key to reach in and unlock their ability to connect with calcium.

In fact, the entire clotting process is extremely complex and involves many more steps and chains of events than those described here. It's a fascinating research topic. However, the steps described here were chosen because they enable us to understand how vitamin K1 and calcium are related to the platelets and the coagulation cascade.

We also noticed the connection between vitamin K1 and K2: they are both intimately involved in calcium metabolism, giving different proteins the ability to connect with calcium. With this knowledge, we are much better equipped to understand the functions of vitamin K2 and will never again confuse it with vitamin K1.

Why is the blood clotting process so complex, requiring so many steps?

Because clotting is a dangerous process. If your blood clots in the wrong place it may cause the blockage of a vital blood vessel, killing you. But, if blood has reached the surface of your skin, then, of course, it needs to clot, for if it is in contact with the oxygen in the air, that's a clear sign there's a tear in your skin. In a nutshell, to coagulate *out* of the body, the blood no longer requires so much paperwork — a real feat of biochemical engineering, don't you agree?

Suppose now that you *don't* want the blood to clot — what do you do? You need to interfere with some of the steps involved in clotting.

A drug called warfarin does just that. Warfarin affects the reuse of vitamin K1,[101] reducing our clotting ability. This is beneficial because it further reduces the likelihood of a blood clot forming in the wrong place. Usually, this medication is given to prevent strokes — cerebrovascular accidents (CVA). At the same time, this drug comes with significant side effects. Why? Because by impairing vitamin K1 metabolism it also impairs clotting where it *needs* to occur.

Could it be a smarter way to prevent clotting *only* in places where it *shouldn't* occur?

As noted, in addition to vitamin K1, calcium is also an essential part of clotting. Calcium is involved in "waking up the doorkeeper" — the scramblase — and in connecting the vitamin K1 dependent proteins with the "table" of phospholipids. Without calcium, there's no coagulation. In fact, if you don't want blood to clot outside of the human body, you just need to join citrate. Citrate reacts with calcium forming calcium citrate thereby rendering coagulation impossible.[102]

Now, our goal is to move calcium away from certain places — the wrong places. How can we do this? Oh, if only there was a molecule capable of moving calcium away from soft tissue! A molecule that, simultaneously, helped calcium to go to where it's needed. Well, we know that this molecule exists, don't we? It's called vitamin K2.

We now understand how vitamin K2 directly relates to cardiovascular disease. Vitamin K2 helps in removing calcium deposits from arteries. Why is this so significant?

Because, as stated in the introduction of this chapter: "the buildup of calcium in the arteries feeding the heart is one of the major risk factors [for heart disease]." This means the more calcium you have accumulated in your coronary arteries, the greater your chances of some blood ending up clotting there, causing you to suffer a heart attack.

How does vitamin K2 perform its function?

Just like vitamin K1 activates clotting factors, vitamin K2 actives osteocalcin. And just like activated clotting factors glue themselves to calcium, so does activated osteocalcin. Except that osteocalcin it's present in the tissues where calcium should be, acting like a magnet, pulling up calcium deep into the bone tissue. For this reason, vitamin K2 has a remarkable role in the health of our skeleton.

Vitamin K2 is the key to understand why so many people supplement with calcium without success. Moreover, if you have osteoporosis and you aren't taking vitamin K2, calcium supplements may even be harming you, because calcium will be more likely to end up being deposited in the wrong place. Of course, if you take high doses of vitamin D you don't need to supplement with calcium since vitamin D is already helping your intestines in absorbing *too much* calcium.

Additionally, vitamin K2 attenuates the bone mineral loss promoted by vitamin D. Along with exercise, vitamin K2 also stimulates our bones to absorb calcium.

Therefore, by joining vitamin K2 to our basic regimen of vitamin D, magnesium chloride and vitamin B2, we'll be doing a favor to our arteries, our kidneys and our bones. What a wonderful vitamin!

Sources of Vitamin K1

In humans, vitamin K1 has a close relationship with calcium and the coagulation process. What about in plants? In the vegetable kingdom, the function of this same molecule is much different. In plants, vitamin K1 is involved in photosynthesis, a process that uses sunlight and carbon from the air to essentially build glucose. For this reason, where can we expect to find vitamin K1? In all that it is green, especially green leafy vegetables.

Most people are not deficient in vitamin K1 because it is present in the green vegetables that most of us frequently eat.

Sources of Vitamin K2

Vitamin K2, on the other hand, it's much more difficult to acquire through diet. Although it's found in meat from animals raised outdoors and fed on fresh grass, it's present in small quantities.

The yolk of an egg from chickens raised outdoors and allowed to feed on the green grass, for example, also contains vitamin K2. The major sources of this vitamin, however, are foods fermented by bacteria like Gouda cheese[103] and Natto, a traditional Japanese food made from fermented soybeans which is, perhaps, the largest natural source of vitamin K2.[104]

When was the last time you saw someone eating Natto? Or worrying — and having the financial means — to feed regularly on meat, eggs and cheese from certified organic farms? No wonder then, that most of us are deficient in vitamin K2. Due to this, our body has a hard time moving calcium away from soft tissue and into bones and teeth — even despite its ability to convert some vitamin K1 into vitamin K2.

What kind of vitamin K2 should you be taking?

If you do an *online* search, you'll find there are several types of vitamin K2, like MK-4, MK-7 and MK-9, with vitamin K2 MK-4 and vitamin K2 MK-7 being the most used in the supplementation industry.

What do these numbers mean?

Pay close attention to the following diagram.

This image perfectly illustrates the structural similarity between vitamin K1 and vitamin K2. In addition, it shows us where the numbers 4 and 7 come from. How?

To understand that, we must first understand what all these lines and hexagons in the image mean. This requires a brief introduction to the fascinating world of organic chemistry.

What is organic chemistry?

In nature, the function of a molecule isn't determined only by what atoms it contains. Of equal importance is how these atoms are structured together. For example, the same number of carbon atoms can give origin to a diamond or to graphite.

The carbon atoms look the same, however, the substances they have formed are very different. Diamond is hard and valuable. Graphite is soft, fragile and, by comparison, of little commercial value. Why this difference? Because, in each case, carbon atoms are connected differently.

Imagine that a carbon atom — represented by an uppercase "c" — is a person with four arms.

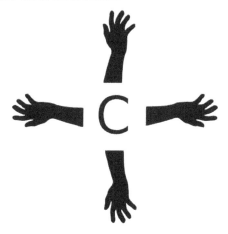

If we add two of these carbon atoms, how will they hold hands? They have several options. For example, they can choose to hold just one of each other's hand. In this case, each of them will have three free hands remaining:

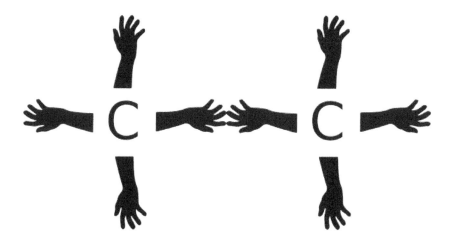

Or they can choose to hold two of their hands together. If they do so, they will now have two connections between them and two free hands each:

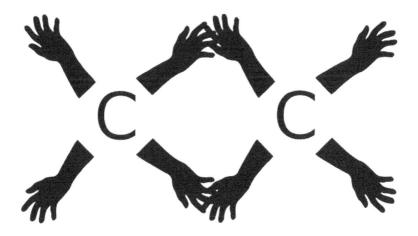

Now imagine we put several of these carbon atoms together. Depending on how they choose to grab each other's hands, they can end up forming a strong structure — like a diamond — or fragile structure — like graphite.

It turns out that carbon is the basis of organic molecules. Why? Because carbon can be used to build a chain and each atom will still be left with two free hands. For example, suppose we place eight carbon atoms, side by side, in a row. Each will still have two free hands for holding other atoms. Moreover, the carbon atom in each corner will have three free hands left, as the following image illustrates.

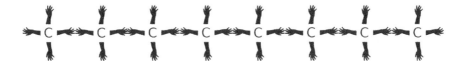

Usually, free carbon hands tend to be holding hydrogen atoms. Hydrogen atoms only have one arm. This means hydrogen works as nature's placeholder. Therefore, our molecule with eight carbon atoms, in reality, would look like this:

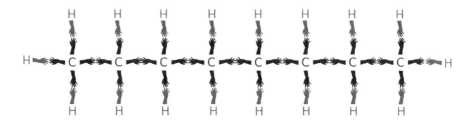

The chemical formula of our substance would be C_8H_{18}. This substance actually exists and is called octane.[105]

The discipline that analyzes the structure of molecules is called organic chemistry. If you go to google images and search the name of any molecule you will eventually find a picture of its chemical structure. However, often you will not find the "C" nor the "H." Why? For the sake of simplicity.

For example, returning to our example of eight carbon atoms and eighteen hydrogen atoms, the octane molecule would normally be represented as:

Why?

Because we know that carbon is always present, forming the skeleton of organic matter. Also, we know that hydrogen is the placeholder of choice. So, to simplify things, it's like if one day scientists got together and decided they would only draw the links between carbon atoms without putting a "C" there. After all, the whole world would know it could only be a carbon atom at each connection point. At the same time, the placeholder — the hydrogen atom — wouldn't also be drawn because everybody would know that if carbon has free arms with no letters attached, then it's because these arms are grabbing hydrogen.

Perhaps you are wondering why the line isn't straight. The answer is that if the line was straight you wouldn't notice where each part of the structure begins and ends.

Compare:

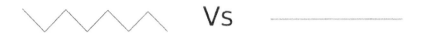

In fact, a straight line would represent C_2H_6 — or ethane.[106] The following image shows us what a scientist would think if he saw a straight line:

Ethane

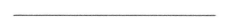

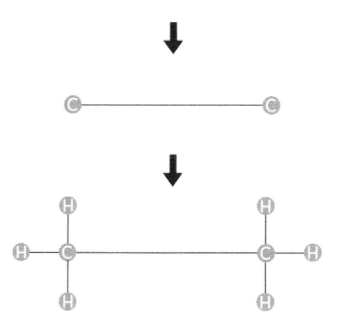

Therefore, you can't just draw a straight line, unless you are drawing ethane.

Now, note how all the following diagrams represent the same substance, from the simplest to the most complex. Also, pay attention to how the complexity of the image increases rapidly as we add details to it until it becomes very hard to have a quick perception of the atomic composition of the molecule:

Octane

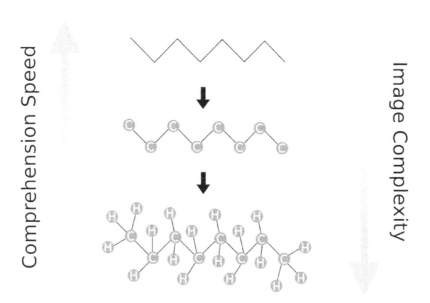

To conclude our brief introduction to organic chemistry, we need to understand just one more aspect. As you can imagine, in nature, certain carbon structures arise very often. One of them is a hexagon characterized by its alternating double bonds:

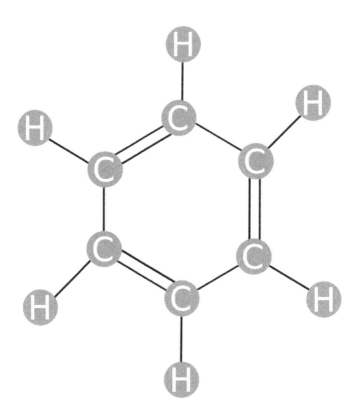

Again, and to make things easier, scientists decided to give names to these structures. This is useful because it allows a scientist to communicate clearly with others. This hexagon is called a benzene ring.[107]

Benzene Ring

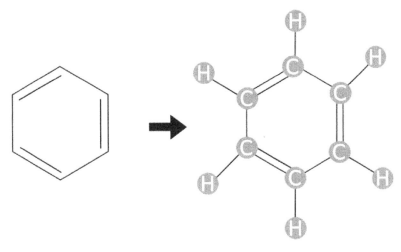

Now that we have a basic understanding of organic chemistry, we are ready to look once again at our molecules of vitamin K:

K1

MK-4

MK-7

We notice that at the beginning there's a familiar structure: It's a hexagon similar to a benzene ring but connected to a second ring which has two oxygen atoms. Oxygen has two available connections — two arms — and both connections in each oxygen atom are attached to its respective carbon atom. This set of two rings has a name: methylated naphthoquinone ring. Next to it comes what seems a long tail. It's only here at the tail that we finally see the fundamental difference between vitamin K1 and vitamin K2 MK-4. Can you see what it is?

In its tail skeleton, Vitamin K1 has just one double bond, followed by single carbon bonds. The MK-4 molecule, however, has four double bonds in its tail. At the same time, the image clearly shows us the difference between MK-4 and MK-7. It's in the number of double bonds in the tail. The MK-4 molecule has four of these double bonds, but the MK-7 version has seven.

This tail consists of structures that are a waste product of the vitamin construction process. In MK-4 the waste structures are repeated four times and, in the MK-7, seven times. It follows that in MK-9 it would be repeated 9 times.

From all the vitamin K2 versions, MK-4 and MK-7 are the most interesting to us because of their effect on the human body.

Which of the K2 vitamins should you choose to supplement with? MK-4 and MK-7?

Scientific studies have shown the MK-7 version has a higher absorption rate and remains active for longer periods of time in the human body.[108] At the same time, some users in online forums report they felt greater benefits with the MK-4 version. However, it is quite difficult to assess the veracity of opinions found in discussion boards. It's not that people are lying, but nothing assures us that they are doing an adequate assessment of what is going on with them.

To exemplify, common comments include: "Vitamin Z[109] is great! I started taking vitamin Z and I haven't had the flu for more than a year. In addition, I am also supplementing with curcumin and manuka honey, among other things."

Although it's easy to read such a comment and get excited about the idea of taking "vitamin Z" for flu prevention, how can we know for sure? Was it vitamin "Z" or one of the other supplements? In fact, good results may even have been obtained by the power all the supplements combined or any other factor not specified. Given this uncertainty, how could we come to a conclusion? We would have to analyze the scientific studies linking flu with each of these supplements. At least by doing so, we would understand if any of them could be of benefit to us.

Therefore, with respect to the debate between MK-4 and MK-7, we must consider that this is a recent field of research, so it's normal for some people to report different results from what those few scientific studies seem to indicate. The truth is the number of studies establishing the superiority of MK-7 against MK-4 are much smaller than, for example, the volume of studies demonstrating the benefits of supplementing with vitamin K2.

Thus, instead of being paralyzed, not knowing which of the two versions to take, the ideal would be to choose both. As described before, one of the vitamin K2 supplements commonly sold contains 200 micrograms of vitamin K2 MK-7 along with 1,000 micrograms of vitamin K2 MK-4.[110]

To end our consideration on vitamin K it's important to note that our intestinal flora also plays an important role in the metabolism of this molecule, so it's important to take good care of our intestinal bacteria.[111] A probiotic, like kefir or another one available in capsule form, will be of help.

Be careful, however, with probiotics purchased online. There are important variations from manufacturer to manufacturer, but some probiotics bottles must be kept refrigerated or else bacterial populations will suffer. This means that one of those bottles, if sent via postal mail or via a common carrier, may arrive at your home in a deteriorated condition.

In the following section of our book, we will be analyzing in more detail the role of vitamin D and vitamin K2 in various pathologies. Starting with depression.

Important warning

It's worth mentioning again the previous warning: Due to the close relationship between vitamin K2 and vitamin K1, **if you are taking anticoagulants you absolutely need to consult your doctor before taking vitamin K2.** Also, if you are taking the pill[112] or any other drug with an associated risk of clot creation you should consult with a doctor before supplementing with either vitamin K1 or K2. This extra layer of safety will assure you the best of results in the safest manner.

Do you remember?

Questions

A.   What is the function of vitamin K1?

B.   What is the relationship between vitamin K1 and calcium?

C.   What is the function of vitamin K2?

D.   What is the relationship between vitamin K2 and calcium?

E.   What is the difference between vitamin K2 MK-4 and vitamin K2 MK-7?

Answers:

A. Vitamin K1 is an essential molecule in the blood clotting cascade. It has a format that fits the clotting factors and modifies them to allow them to attach to calcium. It's as if vitamin K were a master key, and each of the coagulation factors had a lock requiring vitamin K to come in to unlock some of their functions.

B. Vitamin K1 activates the calcium binding property of coagulation factors. Without the action of vitamin K1, coagulation factors would be unable to remain on the surface of the phospholipid table.

C. Vitamin K2 is responsible for activating osteocalcin and MGP, allowing them to interact with calcium.

D. Osteocalcin is present in bones and teeth and MGP is present in soft tissues. When vitamin K2 activates MGP, this causes calcium to leave our soft tissues. When vitamin K2 activates osteocalcin, this causes calcium to bind to our bones. Thus, vitamin K2 acts as a calcium carrier of sorts, removing calcium from where it shouldn't be and taking it to where it's needed.

E. The difference is in the source and format of the molecule. Vitamin K2 MK-4 is found mainly in animal products. Vitamin K2 MK-7 is found in foods that suffered bacterial fermentation. Due to their differences in format, vitamin K2 MK-7 is better absorbed and stays detectable in the human body for longer periods of time.

Section 3

Digging Deeper
Into the Benefits

Chapter 8

Is Vitamin D
Superior to Antidepressants?

"The human brain has 100 billion neurons, each neuron connected to 10 thousand other neurons. Sitting on your shoulders is the most complicated object in the known universe."

— Michio Kaku, Scientist

Depression involves the most complex object in the universe. What could be of help?

When you search for the terms "vitamin D3 + Depression" in the National Library of Medicine, looking for an association between the two, you get more than 200 results.[113] This already tells us that there's probably a link between the two. After all, if this link didn't exist, we would find fewer results, possibly only a handful of studies stating that there's no relevant association between vitamin D and depression.

Why could it there be a link between the two?

Do you remember the instruction booklet analogy used in the first chapter? We explored the relationship between hormones and cells and observed that when activated vitamin D came into contact with the cell it changed the way that cell operated.

It turns out that vitamin D is a hormone that also regulates how our body handles stress. Specifically, among its many other regulatory functions, vitamin D helps our body to utilize at least four of the hormones involved in depression: adrenaline, noradrenaline, serotonin and dopamine.

To understand more fully the beneficial effects of vitamin D on depression, we'll analyze more thoroughly the role of each of these hormones on the onset and maintenance of the depressive state.

Adrenaline and depression

Adrenaline is one of the chemicals responsible for regulating the state of emergency of our body. As already explored at the beginning of this book, adrenaline transforms us into superhumans. How?

Under its influence, our body shuts down its less essential functions and focuses mainly on providing energy to our muscles. Why would this be useful in an emergency?

Imagine you have to flee from a lion. What should be your priority: digesting food or sending the extra blood feeding the stomach cells to the muscles of your legs so that you could run faster? This is why, when under too much stress, our belly aches:

adrenaline puts the brakes on digestion. Simultaneously, our heart rate increases. Why?

We don't notice it, but while our heart is racing, our liver is responding to adrenaline by flooding the blood with extra energy in the form of fat and glucose. Furthermore, our breathing rate has increased, and this caused more oxygen to enter our bloodstream. This nutrient–rich blood needs to get to our muscles as soon as possible, and that's why our heart is beating faster.

However, as you can imagine, adrenaline causes great stress on the entire organism. After all, there's a reason why we aren't always in superhuman mode: the tremendous wear and tear it causes on our system. This is similar to what happens with an overclocked computer processor (CPU).

Some computers have very powerful processors, capable of operating at a higher speed than factory settings allow for. Some computer enthusiasts know how to unlock this extra capacity, in a process called overclocking. But there's a reason why the manufacturer capped the CPU power: the higher the speed, the hotter a CPU gets. Because of this, some of these enthusiasts end up frying their CPUs.

Similarly, our body isn't prepared to *always* work with superhuman mode switched on. Quite the opposite.

Under normal circumstances a lion would appear, our body would activate the superhuman mode and we would run away. Once our brain realized the lion was sufficiently far away, it would switch the emergency mode off. As a direct result, adrenaline levels would drop, and we would enter a state of relaxation and recovery. In this relaxed state, our body would have the opportunity to repair the damage caused by the preceding surge of adrenaline.

Unfortunately, in real life, some problems tend to not disappear. No matter how much you flee from them, you look back and the lions are still there. Perhaps you are facing financial problems or you, or a loved one, are suffering due to a serious illness. These are difficult problems to resolve. It's perfectly normal to feel anxious about them.

Your brain looks at these problems as lions from which it needs to protect you from. So, the brain commands your body to produce adrenaline. Your brain is trying to help you by giving you the necessary extra strength to either run or fight. But most problems can't be solved by running or by fighting. What happens then?

The extra adrenaline keeps you awake at night, turning in bed, your heart beating hard, while you try to fall asleep. Your body is in superhuman mode — an exhausting state of emergency — but you can't escape from the problem, therefore emergency mode remains active day after day, night after night, wearing down on you.

Over the weeks your body begins to show you the signs of mental and physical exhaustion. This mental fatigue, caused by the depletion of your mental stamina, literally modifies the chemical composition of your brain. Eventually, you begin to feel sad and discouraged, unable to regain your lost mental energy and the sense of hope you previously had: you are beginning to feel depressed.

And now you're in a vicious cycle: The problems that caused the initial activation of the stress response are still there and now, they are joined by this new preoccupation with the sadness and discouragement you are feeling daily. And with this new concern arises a new attempt, even more intense, from your brain to help you. And how does your brain try to help? By commanding the release of more adrenaline, intensifying the state of emergency — the very state that already wore your brain down to the point where it can no longer function correctly. What a problem!

Soon enough and your mental and physical energy reserves become so low you sink into a state of deeper depression, a vicious cycle that makes people long for any escape, even suicide. How could there be anything able to help? In a moment we will see.

Serotonin and Depression

Serotonin is the chemical responsible for controlling the importance we give to things. How? Imagine a young man who has just met a girl. They talk for a while and he really enjoys it. After he's back home, what happens? He can't stop thinking about her.

Why? Because his brain is behind the scenes orchestrating things, making him unable to stop wondering what to do next to meet her again. How? By lowering his serotonin levels.6

The boy lays down and can't stop thinking about the girl. "Should I call her? Send her a message? Or wait?"

When serotonin brain levels drop we become obsessed, we can't stop ourselves from ruminating on the subject.

Serotonin is one of the chemicals modified during the activation of the stress response. But, how is serotonin related to the superhuman mode?

Imagine a hungry tiger is chasing you. Is it useful to be relaxed and thinking about other matters? Imagine the tiger is just a few meters away from you and your brain is thinking about your plans for the next day. That would be catastrophic.

If the tiger is coming after you, you must focus on what's going on, the emergent danger. This is accomplished by dropping serotonin. By doing so, your brain makes sure you stay focused on the problem, until it's resolved, no matter how long this takes.

Notice how this is very similar to what happens in depression?

When you are depressed, and you are lying in bed, trying to fall asleep, your neurotransmitters and hormones are trying to accomplish something completely different. Adrenaline increases, keeping you awake, preparing your body to get up and attack the problem head-on. At the same time, serotonin remains low forcing you to stay focused on the problem until it's resolved.

That's why when you are depressed it's difficult to stop thinking about the problems you wish to forget.

Of course, all this is another vicious cycle. The more you think about it the more your brain believes you are in danger and the more it activates the emergency mode. This is just another reason why depression is a *real* disease. The chemical changes occurring in your brain are as real as any other bodily process. Unfortunately, it's not just about adrenaline and serotonin. At least two other chemicals will become deregulated as depression deepens.

Norepinephrine and depression

Ever heard of psychomotor retardation? Even you have never heard this technical term, you certainly have observed its effects. When a person is suffering from depression, lack of energy is a common complaint. Not your regular tiredness, but a pervasive loss of strength that transforms even the simple act of picking up dirty clothes off the floor into a real struggle. Sometimes depression comes to a point where a person doesn't even have the strength to get out of bed. In addition, the depressed person will complain his mind seems to be working more slowly. Why is this happening?

For our muscles and our brain to perform their functions, they need a countless amount of chemicals in the right proportions. Do you recall the sheer complexity of the coagulation process? Then just imagine the complexity of our muscles and brain! One of these chemicals is norepinephrine.

What happens is that superhuman mode eats away our norepinephrine reserves and, without norepinephrine, there's no capacity for movement or thought. Functioning with low levels of norepinephrine is a demanding task. Trying to bend down to pick up clothes from the floor becomes as difficult as bending down to pick up a 100 kg weight.

But why isn't our body turning off the state of emergency? Why force the body into such a state of energy decay?

Well, again, imagine you are being chased by an animal, this time a cougar. Suppose you have norepinephrine reserves to keep the state of emergency active for 30 minutes.

For 30 minutes you can run away from the cougar. After 30 minutes sirens begin ringing inside your brain. Brain cells start telling each other that the norepinephrine levels are getting too low. Imagine that you are now the brain's commander-in-chief. You have two options: keep the emergency mode turned on or ordering it to be shut down. Let's explore each of these possibilities.

Imagine you choose to switch the emergency mode off. Well, that's good because it allows the body to enter a state of recovery. With the superhuman mode turned off, adrenaline levels drop and your heart frequency and breathing patterns normalize. Your stomach restarts digestion. Serotonin increases again, and you can ignore the immediate threat posed by the cougar and think about the movie you saw last night. And the best of all is that you saved your norepinephrine reserves, so you can rest assured: you will continue to have enough norepinephrine to pick up dirty clothes off the floor. There's just a small issue: you became cougar lunch...

Your second option involves maintaining the superhuman mode active. In this case, your body will give everything it has to get away from the cougar. Of course, you have passed the 30 minutes limit, so your muscles won't work as well as before, your brain might begin to process things a bit slower. Maybe your running speed decreases a few percentage points but at least you still have a surviving chance.

Your muscles are getting filled with lactic acid. Lactic acid is a substance that our muscles produce when they are working hard. As lactic acid accumulates you feel the pain. Your whole body is on the verge of collapse. This is when your body plays another trump card: it alters the levels of substance P, a hormone related to the perception of pain. It's as if your body decided to shut down your ability to feel pain. And you keep running.

Will you escape the cougar? We don't know. But one thing is for sure: keeping superhuman mode switched on is still your best option.

Did you notice how strikingly similar this whole process is to depression? When we are facing problems we can't solve — problems that our brain sees as very serious — our brain is set up to keep superhuman mode switched on, even if this means consuming our norepinephrine reserves.

Dopamine and depression

One of the basic characteristics of depression is the difficulty to feel pleasure. When we aren't depressed it's easy to feel delighted. A lively conversation about a topic we love, a good movie, even a beautiful landscape — all these things cause the release of dopamine in our brain.

Dopamine is the chemical of pleasure. You know those hard drugs that people have an immense difficulty quitting, like cocaine? These drugs activate dopamine receptors. In the beginning, they make the person feel intense pleasure, that's why they are so addictive. And what happens when you take the person off the drug? Her brain collapses. The drug damaged the person's brain chemical balance so bad that until he allows time for this balance to be restored, his pleasure centers will be crying for cocaine.

It turns out that, when you go into depression, not only serotonin and norepinephrine are affected, so does dopamine. That's just one more reason why depression is such a painful disease.

Having depression means you have your superhuman mode active, even when your body is no longer able to allocate the necessary resources to remain in superhuman mode.

Returning to the computer example, having depression is like if you forced the processor to continue working even after the circuit had begun to melt.

Of course, the adrenaline and the stress it originates are not the only causes of depression. Often, other problems directly affect the levels of dopamine, norepinephrine and serotonin. For example, if you have thyroid problems this will affect your entire body and may cause depression.

This is why depression is such a complicated disease to treat. Could the super hormone come to our aid? Ultimately, what's the role of vitamin D in all this?

Vitamin D and depression

As it turns out, vitamin D is a modulator of the hypothalamic-pituitary–adrenal axis, regulating epinephrine, serotonin, norepinephrine and dopamine.[114]

It's like if, without enough vitamin D, our body gets confused and finds it troublesome to properly regulate the production of these other hormones and neurotransmitters.

In other words, activating the stress response is a very bureaucratic process. Inside your brain, there are various organelles responsible for assessing the surrounding danger and deciding whether activating the stress response it's worth it or not. In addition, there are several glands involved.

A gland is an organ responsible for producing hormones.

All these organs, ranging from the brain to the adrenal glands, form a kind of vertical line or axis. It's precisely this axis that vitamin D has the ability to influence.

All these organs have vitamin D receptors, or, in other words, all of them have special features that only vitamin D can unlock.

These functions include a protection circuit against dopamine and serotonin depletion.

In addition, vitamin D is directly associated with how our body *uses* stress hormones and the chemicals responsible for feelings of pleasure.

With this in mind. What do the clinical studies reveal about the effect of vitamin D on depression?

In *Vitamin D and Depression: A Systematic Review and Meta-Analysis Comparing Studies with and Without Biological Flaws*,[115] a group of researchers got together to make an analysis of the many scientific studies examining the relationship between vitamin D and depression.

This is called a "meta–analysis" as the Greek word "meta" indicates since it means "beyond." In other words, the researchers went beyond the individual clinical studies, looking for the emergent patterns. What did they find in this meta-analysis?

They found many biological studies had flaws. This means the studies could have been carried out using, for example, insufficient amounts of vitamin D, among other problems.

However, as the meta-analysis found out, studies using adequate amounts of vitamin D obtained good results.

When these researchers focused on properly conducted studies, their conclusion was: "Meta-analysis of studies without biological flaws demonstrates that **improving Vitamin D levels improves depression** (...)" *(Emphasis added)* and: "the effect size of Vitamin D demonstrated in our meta-analysis may be comparable with that of antidepressant medication.

(...)

Should these results be verified by future research, these findings may have important clinical and public health implications."

What dose of vitamin D was used? By analyzing the various studies, these researchers found out that dosages ranged between 400 IU and 18,400 IU.

However, as analyzed in chapter 6, the doses of vitamin D routinely practiced by physicians involved in experimental protocols are of 1,000 IU per kilogram of body mass of the person being treated (1,000 IU per 2.20 pounds).

No wonder then, that these physicians are getting such positive results, especially since their protocols include other supplements with antidepressant effects, like magnesium[116] and vitamin B12.[117] And all this without the side effects associated with antidepressants.

Of course, if you are taking antidepressants, you can't just stop taking them altogether and replace them with vitamin D without your doctor's authorization. Ideally, you should look for a knowledgeable doctor, expert in the use of vitamin D, or show the clinical studies cited here to your current doctor. This is especially important because, for example, a study examining the coadministration of vitamin D and fluoxetine — a serotonin reuptake inhibitor used in the treatment of depression — obtained good results.[118] Therefore, a qualified doctor may decide you will benefit more from a coadministration of vitamin D and an antidepressant.

Still on the topic of dosing, a study evaluating the relationship between supplementation with vitamin D and seasonal affective disorder — a type of depression caused by insufficient sunlight — doses in the order of 100,000 IU were administered, obtaining excellent results in the face of the other common treatment options for seasonal affective disorder, like phototherapy.[119]

Therefore, we must ask: What if researchers had used similar high doses with regular depression instead of just 18,400 IU? Hopefully, studies of this caliber will soon see the light of day.

What about vitamin K2?

Although there are still no studies in humans, there are encouraging reports on the effect of vitamin K2 on anxiety and depression in laboratory animals.[120] This means that vitamin K2 has, at least, the potential to act as an anxiolytic in humans. In any case, by the fact that vitamin K2 allows us to increase the safety of high doses of vitamin D, vitamin K2 can always ensure its presence in any protocol involving vitamin D.

In the next chapter, we will analyze the relationship between vitamin D and autism.

Do you remember?

Questions:

A. What is the stress response?

B. What is the relationship between depression and...
    a. ...adrenaline?
    b. ...serotonin?
    c. ...norepinephrine?
    d. ...dopamine?
    e. ...vitamin D?

C. What were the vitamin D doses used in clinical studies and with what result?

Answers:

A. The stress response is an emergency mode designed to transform our body into a fleeing or fighting machine, a sort of superhuman mode. Several hormones and neurotransmitters work together so that our bodies place any non-essential processes in standby, while at the same time prioritizing survival related mechanisms.

B. The relationships are as follows:

    a. Adrenaline is one of the hormones responsible for the activation of the stress response. Under the effect of adrenaline, our heart beats faster, our breathing rate increases, and nutrient-rich blood and oxygen are diverted from the stomach, and other momentarily non-essential organs, towards the muscles to increase our chances of survival. If the stress response remains active for too long it will cause the depletion of our body's resources and deregulate serotonin, dopamine and norepinephrine levels, causing a negative effect felt strongly on the brain.

    b. Serotonin controls our ability to obsess on a subject. Low levels make us get caught in a subject. High levels help us relax. In depression, serotonin drops, making it difficult for us to stop thinking about our problems.

    c. Norepinephrine is essential for the proper functioning of the nervous system. When its levels drop, thinking and moving becomes harder. A point may come where simple movements seem colossal tasks. Low enough norepinephrine levels are responsible for the onset of psychomotor retardation. Really low levels of this key chemical can render a person unable to get out of bed. All these are typical symptoms of deep depression.

d. Dopamine is the chemical of pleasure. When a person enters a state of depression he will have a hard time feeling any pleasure, this is because the metabolism of dopamine is affected by the underlying root causes of depression.

e. Vitamin D has the ability to modify the whole axis of organs and glands responsible for the activation and management of the stress response and of our hormones and neurotransmitters. Thus, vitamin D plays a fundamental role in the development and treatment of depression.

C. In clinical studies, doses of vitamin D varied between 400 and 18,400 IU. The results observed showed that vitamin D had at least the same effect as antidepressants — without the side effects.

Chapter 9

Vitamin D and Autism

"I think that autistic brains tend to be specialized brains. Autistic people tend to be less social. It takes a ton of processor space in the brain to have all the social circuits."

— Temple Grandin, Professor of Animal Science, Educator and Autism Spokesperson

A few decades ago autism was almost unheard of. However, in recent years, autism has gained increasing recognition. Nevertheless, few people understand what is involved in this condition. As the above quote shows, autism has everything to do with how the brain has had its neural circuits organized during development.

In the case of Asperger's syndrome, it seems the brain is more suited to the processing of technical information than to the processing of contextual dependent emotional information.

In the case of classical autism, a neurological configuration may be so atypical to the point of preventing the affected person from communicating or even interacting with the outside world. Why does this happen?

What is autism?

Our brain consists of billions of cells specialized in information processing. These cells are called neurons. If we imagine the brain is a company,[121] we can think of each member of the company as representing a neuron. And just as each company employee is assigned to a department, so each neuron of our brain belongs to a module.

For example, a large company may have a marketing department, a human resources department, a customer service department and so on. Similarly, our brain has specialized areas to process the sounds we hear, areas specialized in determining whether these sounds come from other humans or from another source and areas specialized in deciphering any verbal messages that these sounds may contain.

In addition, we have another fascinating area, the area responsible for extracting subtle messages from the tone of voice and the facial expressions of others.

For example, imagine you approach someone you know, and you say: "Hello, how are you." This person can answer: "Hi, I'm fine. Thanks." but is he being sincere? It depends. To understand the real meaning of what was said by him, you take notice of the tone of voice used.

If he spoke in a soft and serious tone you know things are *not* okay. Your next question will be: "I see you're not feeling well today, what happened?" And the person will probably begin to tell you all about his horrible day.

However, had this friend of yours spoken in a normal pace, at a higher than normal volume and with an accompanying smile and you'd have thought he was fine.

You didn't even notice it, but within seconds your brain processed all this voice tone and inflection data through several departments. It happened automatically. You didn't have to keep thinking and spending mental energy forcing yourself to interpret the information. Why? Because you don't have autism.

In autism, the brain has developed differently. In the autistic brain, areas related to communication, socialization and emotional processing, among others, don't develop in a common way. Because of this, an autistic brain can't readily process the underlying intentions expressed in a subtle facial expression or in a change in volume or voice tonality.

Autism exists in a spectrum. This means a person can be more or less autistic. How does this work?

For example, someone with a mild form of autism, or Asperger's syndrome, may have an hard time understanding whether a simple, "I'm fine. Thanks," was sincere or not. The brain departments related to voice processing don't work well, so he needs to consciously think about the underlying meaning of the words he heard.

He may take a few minutes comparing this, "I'm fine. Thanks," with other similar phrases he has heard throughout his life.

However, sometimes the autistic person won't have the necessary time to process these underlying meanings. He must risk a reaction. He may decide the person was being sincere and fail to react appropriately.

Why didn't he detect the sad and depressed tone of voice?

The other person sees this as indifference and contempt, concluding that the autistic is cold and uninterested in other people's affairs. This isn't true. What happened was the result of an autistic brain failing to properly process the emotional data hidden in the message.

It's the equivalent of the customer service department of a big company receiving many complaints about the quality of one of their products. As the company fails to react accordingly, customers conclude the company owners don't care about them. However, what's happening is that customer service isn't communicating all the complaints to management. Consequently, management has no real notion of the seriousness of the problem.

But not all autism is like this. Some people suffer from a deeper form of autism. This means the departments responsible for social-emotional information processing and communication are greatly affected.

A person with profound autism may be unable to speak or react to external stimuli.

Turning to the company's illustration again, it's as if the customer service department didn't even exist. So, the complaints aren't even processed, they just accumulate in the mail.

Autism, however, doesn't affect only those areas. It's just that these are the main areas where others take notice of autistic symptoms. What other areas are affected? For example, sensory information processing, such as temperature perception, and the areas related to impulse control, among many others.

At the same time, especially if the autism isn't too severe, areas related to technical processing like musical theory, mathematics, art and design, and comprehension and production of written material, may be highly developed.

This means you can have someone with a milder form of autism, like Asperger's syndrome, who plays piano and composes songs like a musical genius, but who is unable to tell if you are using irony or being sincere.

What causes autism?

There are many theories, but no one knows for sure. However, in recent years, scientists have discovered something extraordinary: the relationship between vitamin D and autism.

If you have autism, supplementation with vitamin D has a good potential to improve your symptoms.[122]

That's not too surprising. We have noted how this super hormone influences nearly every corner of the human body. In fact, it's not too farfetched to wonder that most neurological issues would react positively to vitamin D supplementation. This is certainly the direction clinical studies seem to be pointing to.

Moreover, recent research shows a woman's vitamin D levels during pregnancy have a direct influence on her chances of giving birth to an autistic child.[123, 124]

Therefore, if you, or someone you know, are pregnant or planning to become pregnant, knowing your vitamin D levels and understanding the benefits of supplementation is crucial. Of course, always under proper medical supervision due to the frailty of the developing fetus.

Currently, autism, mild or not, affects 1 in 68 people. Boys are four times more affected than girls.[125] How would these statistics change if all mothers supplemented with an appropriate level of vitamin D during pregnancy?

The administration of any supplement during pregnancy, or to a child, should only be done after checking with a qualified doctor that this can be done safely.

With this in mind, in one of the studies involving women who already had at least one child with autism, the following vitamin D dosages were used:

- 5,000 IU daily during gestation, this dose being in most cases initiated only from the second quarter.

- 7,000 IU per day throughout the entire breastfeeding period. (Note that these 7,000 IU were taken daily by the mother, not by the child).

- If the child stopped drinking the mother's milk, she (the child) would start supplementation with 1,000 IU daily until she was 3 years old.

For example, if the child suckled up to the age of 12 months, that would mean the child would start taking 1,000 IU of vitamin D from that point on and up to the age of 36 months.

After that period, researchers looked at the percentage of children who eventually developed autism. Then, they looked at the probability of these women having an autistic child — remember these are women who already had at least one autistic child.

What was the conclusion?

When a woman who has had a child with autism has another child, there's a 20 percent chance that this new child will develop autism. However, only 5% of the children involved in the study developed autism. That is, of the 19 children involved, only 1 eventually developed autism.[126]

This was a study of small proportions, but it illustrates the potential of vitamin D when administered to the mother during pregnancy and breastfeeding period and to the child after this breastfeeding period ends and up until the age of 36 months.

In another study,[127] 106 children with autism who had blood levels of vitamin D below 30 ng/mL received a daily dose of vitamin D corresponding to 300 IU for each kilogram of body mass (300 IU per 2.20 pounds), but without ever exceeding daily 5,000 IU. 83 children completed 3 months of treatment.

What was the result?

67 of the 83 children who received vitamin D showed improvement in their autistic symptoms.

Why should there be a relationship between vitamin D and autism?

Dr. John J. Cannel from the Vitamin D Council,[128] in one of his papers published in the journal *Medical Hypothesis*,[129] presents some arguments difficult to ignore:

- "The apparent increase in the prevalence of autism over the last 20 years [between 1987 and 2007, when Dr. Cannel published his work] corresponds with increasing medical advice to avoid the sun, advice that has probably lowered vitamin D levels and would theoretically greatly lower activated vitamin D (calcitriol) levels in developing brains."

- "Animal data has repeatedly shown that severe vitamin D deficiency during gestation dysregulates dozens of proteins involved in brain development and leads to rat pups with increased brain size and enlarged ventricles, abnormalities similar to those found in autistic children."

- "Children with the Williams Syndrome, who can have greatly elevated calcitriol [activated vitamin D] levels in early infancy, usually have phenotypes [or characteristics] that are the opposite of autism."

- "Children with vitamin D deficient rickets have several autistic markers that apparently disappear with high-dose vitamin D treatment."

- "Estrogen and testosterone have very different effects on calcitriol's metabolism, differences that may explain the striking male/female sex ratios in autism."

- "Calcitriol down-regulates production of inflammatory cytokines in the brain, cytokines that have been associated with autism."

- "Consumption of vitamin D containing fish during pregnancy reduces autistic symptoms in offspring."

- "Autism is more common in areas of impaired UVB [ultraviolet B radiation, the kind of solar radiation involved in the metabolism of vitamin D] penetration such as poleward latitudes, urban areas, areas with high air pollution, and areas of high precipitation. [this because the cloudy or rainy weather blocks UVB radiation]."

- "Autism is more common in dark-skinned persons and severe maternal vitamin D deficiency is exceptionally common [in] the dark-skinned."

In addition, in another paper published in the same journal, Dr. Cannel talks about how summer seems associated with a reduction in the symptoms of autism in some children, evidencing a potential relationship between the production of vitamin D and the symptoms of autism.[130]

Something like this wouldn't be surprising because of the intimate relationship between vitamin D and brain development and between vitamin D and several other processes involved in autism like the activation and regulation of the stress response.[131]

In any case, the cause of autism is still a topic with many uncertainties and involved in much debate. What practical nuggets of wisdom can we extract from this hypothesis?

Let us see:

1. Supplementing the mother with adequate doses of vitamin D during pregnancy and breastfeeding may benefit the mother and the baby, as long as there are no specific health problems that could put those benefits at risk, like hypercalcemia or a pre-existing renal impairment. These are two problems a regular panel of blood tests could rule out.

2. Supplementing the baby during the first years of his life plays a key role in the healthy development of the child's brain. Even if the child eventually develops autism, this autism is expected to be more moderate, since the effect of vitamin D on the brain involves increasing the body's ability to repair DNA, reducing inflammation, increasing the tolerance to convulsions, increasing the production of

regulatory T lymphocytes, protecting the mitochondria responsible for producing cellular energy, and reducing oxidative stress by promoting the production of glutathione.[132]

3. Adequate levels of vitamin D are beneficial to anyone, regardless of age or health.

4. The need to be careful about taking any drugs that affect the metabolism of vitamin D during pregnancy like antacids and cortisone and its derivatives.

In the next chapter, we will look at the relationship between vitamin D and vitamin K2 and cancer.

Do you remember?

Questions:

A.   What is autism?

B.   What is Asperger's syndrome?

C.   What is the relationship between vitamin D and autism?

Answers:

A. Autism is a disorder affecting the development of the nervous system, including the brain, where several areas, notably those related to socio-emotional processing, don't develop in a typical way. This atypical development manifests itself in the form of atypical behaviors and attitudes. Autism exists on a spectrum, meaning that one can be more or less autistic depending on the severity of their difficulties processing socio-emotional information, among other behavioral and psychological factors.

B. Asperger's syndrome is a mild form of autism, characterized by a brain with difficulties processing nonverbal information. Someone with Asperger's syndrome can be mistakenly assumed to be arrogant or uninterested in others and their feelings.

C. Recent clinical studies have shown that supplementation with vitamin D can reduce the symptoms of autism. Also, recent research shows that if this supplementation is provided to the woman while she is still pregnant, the chances of her child being born with autism decreases.

Chapter 10

Vitamin D and Vitamin K2 Against Cancer

"Growth for the sake of growth is the ideology of the cancer cell."

— Edward Abbey, Author

The diagnosis of cancer is one of the scariest you can receive. My own family was shaken by this diagnosis in 2009, the year my mother was diagnosed with breast cancer. She passed away on April 15, 2017, a date I will never forget.

When we finally found out about vitamin D and begun supplementation we were in 2015 and her cancer had already spread to the bones, including most of the vertebrae, ribs, skull and pelvis, with strong suspicions that it was also present in the liver. These suspicions were later confirmed to be true.

What if my mother had begun supplementating years *before* developing cancer? Would the disease have progressed at the same pace? Would cancer end up developing at all? We can't know for sure. However, current research seems too promising to ignore.

The percentages change from study to study, but overall, the reductions in the probability of getting cancer, when you supplement with vitamin D, are very uplifting. Furthermore, vitamin K2 itself has significant cancer–fighting properties, as we shall see in a moment.

These results are especially relevant when we consider the current statistics. These reveal a frightening fact: It's estimated that cancer will affect one in two men and one in three women in the United States, and it's expected that the number of new cancer cases will almost double by the year 2050.[133] Accordingly, our consideration couldn't be timelier.

We must know: what is cancer and how do vitamin D and vitamin K2 relate to it?

What is cancer?

Cancer is an extremely complex disease and tens of thousands of the brightest minds in the world have devoted their lives to its study. Nevertheless, we still don't have a clear understanding of all that's involved in this disease. Still, overall, cancer is usually divided into 10 basic hallmarks.[134] Thus, we will analyze each of these 10 characteristics and seek to understand their relationship with vitamin D and vitamin K2.

Hallmark 1 — The cell develops the capacity to give itself permission to divide

Our body is formed by cells. These cells have the capacity to divide and form new cells. However, a normal cell divides only upon receiving a specific order to do so. The ability to multiply is just one of many capabilities of a cell. There are specific hormones, the growth factors, responsible for giving this special permission to the cell so that it can multiply itself.

Occasionally, however, a cell begins to multiply without permission. Why does this happen? Due to a mutation in the instructions. In its manual, the cell has a line of code that states: "You can only divide if given permission." But for various reasons, this clear instruction ends up being erased and a new line of code is written in its place: "You can authorize yourself to multiply." Then, the cell begins to produce its own growth factors

This is troublesome. If a cell multiplies without permission, we will end up with two cells. As each of these cells has the same manual that was copied from the parent cell, each of these new cells will also have the ability to authorize itself. Soon we will have four cells, then eight cells, sixteen, thirty-two and so on. If the body fails to stop this madness, in a few weeks we will have a lump, forming deep inside the body — a lump that will continue to grow exponentially as long as there's enough blood serving it.

Fortunately, our body has a few cards up its sleeve. One being growth inhibitory signals. How do they work?

Hallmark 2 — The cell ignores specific orders to stop dividing

The uncontrolled multiplication of a cell is very dangerous. As such, when the body notices that a cell needs to stop dividing, it sends specific messengers to prohibit this behavior. Unfortunately, sometimes the cell gets its genetic code — its manual — damaged to a point where it can no longer recognize the meaning of the messengers being sent by the body. Any growth inhibiting messenger molecules are promptly ignored. The problem is getting worse quickly. What can the body do now?

Hallmark 3 — The cell loses the ability to self-destruct

Our cells are designed with a safety system called apoptosis. Within each cell, there are sensors that continuously evaluate the cell's insides for any signs that the cell is faulty. When a cell is caught giving itself the authorization to multiply, or ignoring external orders to stop multiplying, these alarms are activated. Upon activation, they initiate cell suicide or apoptosis. When apoptosis is activated, the cell dissolves itself within 30 to 120 minutes and any cell remains are cleaned up by the body.

But there's another problem with our cell. Its sensors are not activating as expected. The cell is simply too damaged for the sensors to work properly. What about now?

Hallmark 4 — The cell overcomes its own multiplication limit

Even with their ability to multiply without permission, the cell has a limit. Perhaps you've heard of telomeres. This is the name given to a kind of protection each of our chromosomes possess. Each time a cell divides the telomere shortens. After a few dozen divisions, human telomere gets shorten to the point where a cell can no longer divide.

Scientists believe this is one of the reasons we get older. Our cells reach the multiplication threshold and die. Finding a way to increase the length of the telomeres is one of the greatest goals of anti-aging science, as this would allow us to live much longer.

It turns out that sometimes a damaged cell develops the ability to create a chemical cocktail that prevents its telomeres from shortening. This is as close to cellular immortality as you can get. Imagine, a damaged cell that is multiplying incessantly escaped from suicide and now has found a way to make itself, and each of its daughter cells, immortal. Now what?

Hallmark 5 — The cell convinces the body to feed it with extra food

Even if a cell can create many copies of itself, each of these new cells still needs to be nourished. And as it turns out, the body has a limited number of blood vessels feeding each cell agglomerate. After all, the body expects that there is only one specific number of cells at any given place.

From the body's perspective, if a cell were to multiply without permission this would activate the internal safety systems and lead to apoptosis — cell suicide. And our body knows that when a cell divides, the old cell dies.

Because of all these reasons, the blood vessels feeding any given area provide the cells at that location with just enough nourishment. This limited vascularization happens to be yet another safety barrier against tumor development. It no longer matters if a cell is mortal or immortal. Eventually, even an immortal cell must stop dividing for lack of enough raw materials — such as proteins or energy in the form of oxygen and glucose.

But even this safety mechanism has a way to be exploited by the cancer cell. How?

For example, if I fall and wound myself, my body will have lost some deep skin cells due to the impact. But it wasn't only the cells that have died, the blood vessels that fed them were also damaged. To fix this, the surviving cells surrounding the wounded area will send out an S.O.S. request. In response to this request, the body allows something special to happen.

The body will issue a special permission regarding vascularization. As a result, new blood vessels will be built from existing blood vessels, bringing the necessary nourishment to the new cells. This process of building blood vessels is called angiogenesis.

You are probably guessing what happens next. That's right, one of these immortal cancer cells will develop the ability to trick the body into issuing this special permit. This, in turn, will result in our own body being deceived into building the necessary infrastructure to feed all those hungry immortal cells.

Where there was only one cell, now there are billions! This tumor, as it keeps growing, may end up endangering a person's life. How? If it grows near a vital organ such as the heart or the liver, it might grow to the point of preventing this vital organ from performing its life-supporting functions, causing the person to die.

Also, as a tumor grows it makes pressure against various pain receptors — like a gum abscess pressing on the nerves of an infected tooth. The only difference being that instead of a group of bacteria, you are dealing with a group of abnormal, immortal, and highly undifferentiated cells. And it's all downhill from here.

Hallmark 6 — The cell acquires the ability to leave the tumor site and enter the bloodstream

Things are quickly worsening. Eventually, one of the tumor cells leaves the primary tumor and enters the bloodstream. Our blood feeds our whole body, so the tumor cell may end up invading other organs of the body. When this happens, it's said cancer has metastasized, or spread. Left untreated it's a matter of months — or perhaps years depending on the aggressiveness of cancer — until the person dies.

Four extra hallmarks

Over the years, researchers noted that for a regular cell to evolve and transform to the point of metastasizing and becoming a real threat, it had to develop some more skills than those defined by the 6 hallmarks. So, they defined 4 new extra hallmarks.

As It turns out, besides the safety mechanisms present in every cell — such as the dependency in external growth signals and apoptosis — we also have an external source of protection: our own army of specialized forces — the white blood cells. Some of these white cells have a special function: inspect every cell. If they notice that a cell is behaving in an abnormal way an extermination order is issued by these inspectors and sent to specialized white blood cells who will attack and kill the cancer cell, regardless of everything else.

Unfortunately, these abnormal cancer cells sometimes develop the ability to camouflage their cancerous nature, disguising themselves as normal cells, cheating the immune system and preventing it from recognizing the real threat standing in from of it.

In her studies, my mother used to marvel at the amazing intelligence of the enemy we were facing. She was particularly impressed by this characteristic.

As if not enough, the cancer cell proceeds to release chemicals that attract specific kinds of soldiers, like macrophages and neutrophils. Then, it's as if the cancer cell brainwashed these soldiers, for lack of a better term, convincing them to release growth signals and angiogenesis requests to the body, further tricking the organism into believing there's a genuine need for extra vascularization at the cancer site.

The cancer cell is tricking the immune cells into using the inflammatory process to cancer's own benefit.

These are two of the new hallmarks described by researchers in recent years: The development of the ability to pretend to be a normal cell and the development of the capacity to recruit the immune system.

As if all this weren't enough, a cancer cell is very unstable at a genetic level. It's as if the cell clerks had gone mad and were constantly rewriting the instruction manual. This means each copy is slightly different. Thus, when doctors administer a chemical, it won't kill all the cells because these cancer cells are not all *exactly* alike. Then, the surviving cells, with their genetic immunity to the chemical, will continue to multiply. Over time most of the cells at the tumor site will be of the resistant type.

The development of genomic instability is another hallmark of a cancer cell.

The last hallmark, which is present from the beginning, has to do with a particularity of cancer cells: they depend on glucose to thrive. A normal cell uses oxygen, glucose and ketones to feed itself. Whereas a cancer cell can only use glucose. This has been known for many decades, but now we know this turns out to be very useful to the cancer cell. How?

In the process of converting glucose into energy, the cancer cell produces a lot of extra proteins. These same proteins end up providing the raw materials required to build new cancer cells at a faster rate.

The four stages of cancer

While the agglomerate of abnormal cells remains at a single original site, it's said it is in the first stage. When the cells start increasing in number, even spreading to the lymph nodes — the sewage system of the body — it is said cancer has reached stage two.

The third stage occurs when cancer cells invade adjacent organs. For example, if the mammary cells divide endlessly to the point of reaching and invading the lung, all the while remaining a single tumor.

The fourth stage is defined by the presence of metastases — i.e. when tumor cells begin to invade other organs. At this stage, new sites of cancer develop, formed by cells belonging to the original tumor. Most deaths occur in this final stage. It's the most dangerous stage.

The role of vitamin D

When we read about cancer and the capabilities that a cancer cell can develop, it's easy to become fearful. This is normal.

Cancer is a real enemy of the human race. Also, statistics are not in our favor. If things continue as they are, with a large percentage of people deficient in vitamin D, even more people will end up developing cancer. But everything's not lost yet.

Remember what we mentioned earlier?

It's estimated that vitamin D has the ability to reduce the rate of cancer incidence in many percentage points because of the multiple ways in which it affects the development and proliferation of tumor cells.[135] For example, a promising study cited once in the preface of this book indicates that supplementation with vitamin D can positively influence the odds of a woman having breast cancer in up to 83%.[136] Other studies on the effect of vitamin D in various types of cancer have also shown promising results, such as with colon,[137] prostate[138] and lung[139] cancer, to name a few.

What does this mean?

Let's look closely at the results of that which seems to be the study with the most promising results. Imagine a group of 1,000 women in the United States. The current statistic is that in the coming decades 1 in 3 of these women will have cancer.

Let's assume that all of them will have breast cancer. This means that in a few years 333 of these women will be diagnosed with cancer.

But suppose now, that we could travel back in time and get all these women on vitamin D — according to the daily needs of each one of them. Now, if we were to travel forward in time, how many of them would continue to have breast cancer? According to the statistics, only about 20% of them, or 66.

This means that in 1,000 women, instead of having 333 cases of cancer, or 1 in 3, we would have 66 cases — 1 in 15.

It's true we have made some serious generalizations that just don't happen in real life and it's clear that not all cancers have such a high reduction rate. However, the goal of this mental exercise it's to illustrate the potential of vitamin D. A reduction of 80% is quite encouraging, even if it only applies, in this way, to breast cancer — don't you agree? In addition, there's another factor that we must account for: the aggressiveness of cancer.

If a person supplements daily with the appropriate dose of vitamin D, even if he ends up developing cancer, will that cancer progress at the same speed? Will that cancer be as likely to reach the metastasis stage?

It's true this is a field under investigation, but I believe it wouldn't be too farfetched to presume vitamin D would also influence the rate of development of the cancers that do end up developing, despite proper vitamin D supplementation.

But how does vitamin D exert this effect? To answer this question, we must revisit the hallmarks described above.

Vitamin D, as the super hormone that it is, enters the cancer cell and interferes with its various features. For example, the cell wants to start giving itself the authorization to divide, but vitamin D interferes with this process. Moreover, Vitamin D stimulates the cell to correct its DNA encoding errors.

Imagine the following situation. A woman may have been hit in the chest. Due to this trauma, breast tissue cells were damaged. But this woman takes her vitamin D every single day. Her blood is teeming with the super hormone. As a result, vitamin D stimulates these breast tissue cells to repair themselves instead of allowing them to go on to develop cancerous characteristics.

This includes the repairing of cell suicide mechanisms. So, if the damage is too extensive to be corrected, vitamin D helps the cell activate apoptosis and destroy itself.

If all else fails and a tumor develops, vitamin D can act in an anti-angiogenic manner. This means vitamin D prevents the cancer cell from convincing the body to build extra blood vessels. Thus, the tumor never gets beyond the size of a harmless microtumor. It's like vitamin D forces the cell to correct its wrongdoing.

In addition, vitamin D has a direct effect on the immune system, fortifying it. In this way, the immune system will be more apt to both detect and attack the cancer cell, even before it develops the ability to cloak itself.

In clinical studies, all these anticancer effects were observed even at daily doses between 2,000 and 4,000 IU. However, as argued throughout this book, under proper care, much higher daily doses may be safely utilized.

What about vitamin K2?

Vitamin K2, as a synergistic helper of the super hormone, also plays an important role in fighting cancer. Recent research indicates this vitamin has the potential to affect the ability of the cancer cell to give itself permission to divide and to ignore external signals to stop dividing, among many other anticancer effects.

The way vitamin K2 achieves this is synergistic with vitamin D. It affects both internal and external processes, by modifying the growth factors the cell is sending into the outer cell space. Additionally, vitamin K2 modifies the growth factors receptors present on the cell's surface.

Thus, vitamin D and vitamin K2 cooperate to prevent the cell from multiplying at random.

Vitamin K2 can also affect the process of apoptosis, stimulating various types of cancer cells to commit suicide, among many other benefits.[140, 141, 142, 143, 144, 145]

As if not enough, a key benefit of vitamin K2 in fighting cancer is how this vitamin helps us to increase the daily dose of vitamin D safely — as explored in Chapter 6.

For all this, each of us would do well to include each of these vitamins in our daily supplementation plan.

In the next chapter, we will analyze, in a more concise way, the role of vitamin D and vitamin K2 in several of the more common diseases of our time.

Do you remember?

Questions:

A.   What are the 10 key hallmarks of a cancer cell?

B.   Why do vitamin D and vitamin K2 have such a significant effect on a person's chances of getting cancer?

Answers:

A. A cancer cell has 10 key characteristics:

> a. the development of the capacity to allow itself to divide;
>
> b. the ability to ignore external instructions to stop dividing;
>
> c. the loss of the ability to self-destruct;
>
> d. the development of the capacity to exceed its own multiplication limit;
>
> e. the development of the ability to convince the body to give it more nourishment by means of angiogenesis;
>
> f. the acquisition of the ability to abandon the tumor site and enter the bloodstream;
>
> g. the ability to convince the immune system to help the cancer cells in their growth efforts;
>
> h. the development of the ability to pretend to be a healthy cell;
>
> i. genomic instability, that is, constant genetic mutation;
>
> j. the dependence on the fermentation of glucose as a source of cellular energy, which in turn provides the cancer cell with the necessary raw material to build new versions of itself.

Although all these 10 characteristics may not be present, if the cancer is left untreated, all of them will have the tendency to manifest.

B. Both vitamin D and vitamin K2 affect several of the characteristics that define a cell as cancerous. In addition, they achieve this in a synergistic manner, by exerting their effect in different ways.

Chapter 11

Heart Disease, Osteoporosis and Autoimmunity Were Just the Beginning: Asthma, Type 1 and Type 2 Diabetes, the Flu, the Common Cold, Fibromyalgia, and Chronic Pain — No Stone Is Left Unturned

"The young physician starts life with 20 drugs for each disease, and the old physician ends life with one drug for 20 diseases."

— William Osler, Scientist

In real life there are no superheroes with superpowers to defend us, but vitamin D and its faithful companion, vitamin K2, come close.

Vitamin D acts as a super hormone and, along with vitamin K2, revitalizes the entire metabolism of calcium, having a positive effect on both cardiovascular disease and osteoporosis.

Then, if you want to lower your risks of atherosclerosis what do you need to do? It's critical to move calcium away from your arteries.

Likewise, if you want to increase your bone density and decrease your chances of developing osteoporosis what is the secret? Find a way to move the calcium to where it needs to be.

But what about other common diseases? What does the scientific research reveal to us?

As we have already done with autoimmune diseases in chapter 6, with heart disease in chapter 7 and with osteoporosis, in chapter 1 and later in chapter 7, we will now look at the relationship between our wonder duo and asthma, diabetes, infectious diseases and pain.

Asthma

Asthma is one of the most common respiratory diseases, affecting millions of people. It's characterized by the inflammation of our airways. The airways of someone with asthma are extremely sensitive and easily react to the presence of dust and other particles.

Our respiratory tract is composed of a main tube, called the trachea, which divides into two smaller tubes called the bronchi. The trachea carries the air to the inverted "Y" intersection and then, this air is directed to each of our lungs through two other tubes: the bronchus.

Inside the lungs there are innumerable channels, a large network of smaller and smaller tubules called bronchioles. The latter are connected to tiny sacs called alveoli. In these alveoli, gas exchanges occur between the air we breathe in and the air we will expire. The best known of these gas exchanges involve oxygen and carbon dioxide.

Although our lungs deal primarily with gases, they are also well-prepared to deal with dust and other particles and microorganisms extraneous to the body.

When we inhale these particles, our lungs react by creating a mucus that surrounds the offending particle. After that, this mucus gradually passes through the labyrinth of tubes until it reaches our throat where it can be either spat or swallowed to be consumed by the stomach acid.

Surrounding all this circuit are many muscle fibers. These can contract, triggering a reaction that we call coughing. When we cough, our internal network of tubes is squeezed. This facilitates a faster expulsion of any mucus or offending particles and microorganisms.

In addition, our immune system and the inflammatory process also play a key role in preventing these offenders from reaching the bloodstream or dwelling and multiplying in our airways.

However, sometimes the person develops an extreme sensitivity to the dust particles and microorganisms present in the air. When this happens, the pulmonary safety system becomes hyperactive, like an alarm whose sensor is so sensitive that it is always causing the siren to go off.

When this happens, inflammatory processes and the coughing mechanism are activated too often. This makes it difficult to breathe. As if that were not enough, the person produces more mucus than normal, even to the point of blocking the airways. Because of this, an asthma attack can shut down the air flow and become life-threatening.

How could vitamin D help? As noted, vitamin D has immunomodulatory properties. This means it helps in calibrating the sensitivity levels of our lungs.[146, 147]

Clinical studies demonstrate this effect. One study showed how a monthly dose of 60,000 IU of vitamin D3 — equivalent to 2,000 IU per day — decreased the need for medication and the number of hospital visits in asthmatic children.[148]

However, studies that begin with high doses of vitamin D followed by reduced daily administrations of the vitamin don't always show relevant effects. This indicates our body needs to receive its daily dose of vitamin D, instead of a single dose in one day, followed by a reduced dose in the following days.[149]

What about vitamin K2?

The truth is the number of studies connecting vitamin K2 with asthma is very low. This is consistent with what we have been talking about: the general lack of knowledge about the role of vitamin K2 — an unfortunate situation which is finally coming to a U-turn. Nevertheless, when looking for information about clinical studies, we find a very interesting one, from the 70's. This study demonstrated that vitamin K2 exerted a positive effect on asthma symptoms. Of the 3 groups of patients investigated, over 90% of patients with mild symptoms of the disease saw improvement, as did about 86% of patients with moderate symptoms. In turn, among those with more severe symptoms, 72.7% showed improvement.[150]

The conclusion is encouraging: therapy with our superhero — vitamin D — and his faithful companion — vitamin K2 — had beneficial effects on asthma, even in cases where dosages were much lower than those used in the experimental protocols.

Do you suffer from asthma?

Then, in addition to vitamin D and vitamin K2, pantethine[151] (a vitamin B5 precursor) has also shown the potential to help. Among naturopaths, pantothenic acid (vitamin B5) itself is used instead of pantethine, along with vitamin C.

Diabetes

Diabetes is a brutal disease that can lead to blindness, amputation, and many other serious problems. It's divided into two types: Type 1 and type 2 diabetes. What is the difference between these two types? Let's see.

Our cells are prepared to use glucose — sugar — as fuel. But there's a problem. The glucose molecule is way too large to enter through the normal cell door. Because of this, glucose needs special credentials to gain entrance through the cell membrane.

In simple terms, there's a hormone that acts as a mediator between glucose and the cell. This mediator is a hormone called insulin.

When insulin reaches the cell, it fits into the insulin receptors. At that point, the cell looks at the manual to find out what it should do in the presence of insulin. The manual is very clear: when insulin arrives, this is a sign that the doors must be wide, wide open, so that glucose may enter.

Inside the cell, glucose is converted into energy. Our brain is the main consumer of glucose, but every cell of our body can use it as an energy source.

Where does insulin come from?

Insulin is produced by beta cells. These cells are located in the pancreas. In a healthy organism, everything runs smoothly. The person consumes his food, the digestive process makes the separation between the various nutrients and releases them into the bloodstream. Among these nutrients is glucose.

In turn, beta cells continuously produce the insulin that will allow all that glucose to steadily flow into every cell in the body. Thanks to insulin, the food we consume can easily become a source of cellular energy.

However, sometimes this smooth process begins to roughen up. Instead of entering the cells, glucose begins to accumulate in the bloodstream. This means a simple test of blood glucose levels will register higher than normal levels.

For example, a doctor is often interested in your fasting blood sugar levels. If the test reveals you are between 70 to 99 milligrams of glucose per deciliter of blood (mg/dl), this means you are within the normal range. But if your values are between

100 to 125 mg/dl this is an indication that your body is no longer processing glucose as it should. In turn, if you got values above 126 mg/dl in two consecutive tests you will be diagnosed as diabetic[152] — meaning your body is no longer able to process sugar without help. But, how did this happen?

There are essentially two reasons.

Type 1 Diabetes

Someone with type 1 diabetes suffers from insufficient insulin production. In most cases, this happens because the immune system is attacking and destroying the insulin-producing beta cells. In other cases, the problem may be of genetic origin. In either case, the person is unable to produce this vital hormone and becomes dependent on insulin injections to survive.

Therefore, type 1 diabetes often has an autoimmune origin.

Type 2 Diabetes

Type 2 diabetes happens when our cells stop responding to insulin. How does this happen?

Glucose is present in our blood at all times and beta cells are always producing insulin to move this sugar into cells. However, beta cells don't release all their insulin in one go — they hold some of it as a buffer. And when do they choose to dump their insulin reserves? After we eat.

When the level of glucose in the blood increases dramatically — after a meal — beta cells will release a considerable amount of the insulin they have in reserve. Sometime later, if blood sugar hasn't yet gone down, they'll release the remaining of their insulin reserves.

After this, beta cells are left without insulin. So, what will they do if blood sugar is still higher than it should? They will do their best to keep producing insulin and sending it right into the blood, trying to keep up with the demand.

However, it turns out that our cells tend to become insensitive to insulin if they are always being stimulated by high amounts of it. This means that regular consumption of foods with a high glycemic index — that is, foods that are readily converted to a high amount of glucose — will force our beta cells to release a significant amount insulin more frequently, contributing to cell insulin insensitivity.

But if cells are becoming insensitive, this means beta cells must work harder. They need to produce much more insulin than normal to get the same effect. But this extra insulin will stimulate an aggravation of cell insulin insensitivity. Do you see where we are going? It's a vicious cycle.

The more insulin is produced, the greater the insensitivity of other cells and the greater the insensitivity, the greater the need for our beta cells to produce more insulin. Eventually, our beta cells can no longer keep up with the demand for more insulin. This causes blood sugar levels to go awry.

Rising blood sugar levels damage our whole organism, including beta cells themselves. We enter in yet another vicious cycle.

Although the beta cell is working as hard as it can, it can't meet the demand for insulin because the person is ingesting way too much sugar. So, this extra sugar kills more and more beta cells. This leads to less and less insulin being produced, with what result? Dangerous blood sugar levels for a longer time. Leading to what? More dead beta cells! And the vicious cycle continues.

To make matters worse, when our liver detects low levels of insulin in the blood it assumes this is because glucose levels are also low. After all, in a healthy individual insulin would only fall if beta cells stopped producing it and they would only stop doing so if there wasn't enough sugar in the blood. So, what does the liver do? It releases its blood sugar reserves. The result? We enter a new destructive cycle: Sugar levels rise even more, beta cells die in greater numbers, there's less and less insulin being produced, and the liver continues to interpret this as a warning sign to release more of its sugar reserves!

Now, in the middle of all this, imagine this scenario: often the person will continue to consume sugar. There's no escape type 2 diabetes.

How can vitamin D help?

In the case of type 1 diabetes, since it is often of autoimmune origin, vitamin D supplementation will keep the immune system from directing its powerful attacks against the beta cells. This means that vitamin D supplementation can delay, or if given early enough, even prevent the development of the disease.

For example, a study conducted in northern Finland collected data from more than 10,000 children. One of their findings was that children who took 2,000 IU of vitamin D during the first year of life had less than 80% chance of developing type 1 diabetes.[153]

In the case of type 2 diabetes, there seems to be a direct relationship between blood levels of vitamin D and the body's ability to deal with excess sugar. To put it in simple terms: The higher the levels of vitamin D in your blood, the lower your chances of developing type 2 diabetes.[154]

We don't know how vitamin D helps beta cells, but these cells have vitamin D receptors. This means they have functions that can only be fully performed when they are being stimulated by the super hormone. Studies done on rats have shown that when you remove these vitamin D receptors from beta cells, the animals are no longer able to produce the same levels of insulin as they did before.[155]

And what about vitamin K2?

Those who have diabetes are at higher risk for fractures. Vitamin K2 supplementation reduces this risk.[156]

And what about an effect on the disease itself?

As in the case of vitamin D, researchers observed that vitamin K2 increases a cells' sensitivity to insulin.[157, 158] In addition, it's noteworthy that osteocalcin also acts as a hormone, helping regulate blood glucose levels.[159] Hence, it isn't surprising why research has established a link between vitamin K2 and diabetes through their mutual relationship with osteocalcin.[160]

Therefore, while the volume of research on vitamin K2 isn't as complete as that on vitamin D, both substances reveal their potential for helping in diabetes prevention and management when put to the test.

The common cold and the flu

Shortly after the First World War, a flu epidemic afflicted the globe and ended up taking more lives than the war itself. Nowadays, the flu does not take this number of lives, not even close, but it continues to be responsible for leaving people in bed, unable to work and in suffering. In addition, people who are more fragile — either due to their age or because of a coexisting illness — may even end up getting their lives at risk when infected by one of the various flu strains.

What is the role of vitamin D and vitamin K2 in preventing this disease?

In February 2017, the University of Harvard published an article entitled "Study confirms vitamin D protects against colds and flu." This study consisted of an analysis of more than 11,000 participants from 25 other studies.[161]

In what ways does vitamin D help us fight respiratory infections?

In Chapter 6 of this book, when we look at the role of vitamin D in the inflammatory response, we saw how it helped our immune system calm down, promoting a reduction in the production of cytokines. Now is the time to talk about another beneficial effect of vitamin D on our immune system: the stimulation of the production of antimicrobial proteins.

When our body is invaded by a virus or a bacterium, our white soldiers can produce substances specially designed to destroy such invaders. It's these very substances we are talking about when mentioning antimicrobial proteins.

What is the result of the vitamin D induced stimulus on the immune system?

For example, one study has found that a healthy person is twice as likely to get influenza if their vitamin D levels are low.[162]

And what about vitamin K2? Unfortunately, sufficient information isn't available. However, because vitamin K2 allows for a higher degree of safety when supplementing with vitamin D, this is enough to make it an essential part of our daily supplementation regime.

Fibromyalgia

Fibromyalgia is a dreadful disease. You have intense, strange, and limiting pains. But whoever looks at you says your body looks great. You do the requested examinations and tests and they come out fantastic. You feel like Cassandra from Greek mythology, who always spoke the truth, but no one ever believed her. No matter where doctors look, they can't find anything wrong with you. This is disconcerting.

The day you need stronger painkillers, as regular painkillers no longer have an effect on your pain levels, you end up in the ER being interviewed by a team of psychologists who try to gauge whether you are actually suffering from pain or just trying to get them to prescribe you heavy painkillers — as if secretly you were a drug addict, pretending to be in pain all these years just to get your next dose of opioid analgesics at any cost.

For years, this has been the reality of fibromyalgia for many sufferers.

Fortunately, recognition of the reality of these kinds of diseases and of the suffering inflicted by them has been increasing. This is important because fibromyalgia seems to affect between 2% and 8% of the population.[163] 8% may not sound like much, but it means one in twelve people.

However, because of the invisible nature of this disease, there are no certainties as to the causes.[164] Many researchers believe our own brain is at fault. How? By amplifying the signals it receives.[165] For example, by processing a simple touch as a punch or by relaying a temperature variation as a pain signal.

The means of alleviating suffering, in turn, are increasingly involving stronger and stronger painkillers, with many undesired side effects. Not to mention the fatigue and other symptoms, over which analgesics have no effect.

In this sense, any help is welcomed, even if it's small.

Could the super hormone be of any help?

Yes, especially if you are deficient in it. Studies have shown that vitamin D deficiency is directly related to muscle and skeletal pain.[166, 167, 168, 169]

In addition, some scientists involved in fibromyalgia research believe there's a strong autoimmune component.[170] If this is the case, then high-dose vitamin D therapy is expected to have the potential to halt this disease altogether, significantly relieving the symptoms.

Chronic Pain

In a single month, nearly 20% of people — one in five — report having general pains in their body. 33% — one in three — shoulder pains and up to 50% — one in two people — lower back pain.[171]

Some of these pains persist for much longer than a month. They become chronic pains. Chronic pain greatly affects one's day-to-day life. Even simple tasks can become monumental challenges.

The worst thing is too many times the origin of these pains is unknown. Leaving you with limited options to do something about it. Sometimes the person may end up with a diagnosis of fibromyalgia, but often he doesn't receive any specific diagnosis. He just knows that his body hurts — a lot.

Sometimes these pains are of muscular origin. If this is the case, a massage of the so-called trigger points will provide significant relief.[172]

To find the right spots, just google for the pain location, followed by the expression "trigger points." For example: "https://www.google.com/search?q=**head+pain+trigger+points**" and observe the results in google images. These images are often self-explanatory.

The massage of trigger points involves pressing down and forward, relieving the pressure and repeating the motion from the beginning. These strokes are continued for about 30 seconds and are repeated several times throughout the day. These kinds of strokes cause pain, so they may not be effective in pains caused by true tissue hypersensitivity and may even make them worse, but will be highly effective — even miraculous — in pain caused by the undue contraction of individual muscle fibers.

Sometimes trigger points arise due to other unrelated pains. How come?

For example, if your right leg hurts you may end up overloading the muscles on the left leg, the stabilizing muscles of the spine and so on. If one member suffers, all other members suffer with it.

If you have access to it, a most effective method for dealing with trigger point pain is one that uses a special type of injections administered by a qualified health professional. In fact, the therapeutic benefit comes directly from the needle piercing through the trigger point and not so much from the analgesic drug being administered simultaneously.

What is the role of vitamin D in this type of chronic pain of unknown origin?

Again, there are studies indicating a relationship between vitamin D deficiency and pain. Especially among those who complain from headaches.[173]

In any case, studies involving the role of vitamin D in pain have used comparatively low doses.

Imagine supplementing someone with 2,000 IU per day to see if vitamin D had any effect on his pain levels, compared to putting that person on the right dose he required to actually react to vitamin D.

Doses of this caliber can even reach 200,000 IU in the case of people with severe problems in the absorption and use of vitamin D — for example, someone obese taking corticosteroids and having several genetic problems related to the processing of vitamin D.

For comparison, this would be like giving 10 mg of paracetamol to someone when that person needed at least 1,000 mg to feel some pain relief.

The truth is that vitamin D isn't an analge
hormone that stimulates our body to behave.
vitamin D doesn't take your pain away after
take days, weeks or months. But it will be worth.

After all, if this pain of unknown origin is caused
autoimmune, inflammatory, or other disorder originating in
of the innumerable cellular processes that vitamin D influences,
you will have to feel the difference. It's expected that, at a
minimum, taking a physiologically active dose of vitamin D — the
one which lowers PTH to the recommended minimum values —
will have some effect on these kinds of pains.

After all, if there's any lesson we can draw from the detailed
analysis of these section of the book, it's this: **now that we know
how to administer high doses of vitamin D safely, this should be
one of the first therapeutic approaches in the fight against any
disease that does not involve the safety mechanisms themselves
— like kidney disease.**

Be it the aches, cancer, heart problems, autism, depression,
autoimmune disease or any other type of chronic illness, the steps
we must take are always the same. Therefore, under the
supervision of your doctor, do the other treatments he
recommends, but also start taking vitamin D and assessing your
PTH levels over the months, until they reach the desired
minimum value. Why?

Because at worst you will be giving your body the best chances
to react appropriately to the disease.[174] And this, along with any
other therapeutic approaches, will increase your chances of
beating the disease.

At best you might see your problem entering remission after a
few months.

In the next chapter, we will summarize everything we have
learned throughout our consideration of the role of vitamin D and
vitamin K2 in the human metabolism.

Do you remember?

Questions:

A.   What is asthma?

B.   What is the relationship between vitamin D and asthma?

C.   What is type 1 diabetes?

D.   What is the relationship between vitamin D and type 1 diabetes?

E.   What is type 2 diabetes?

F.   What is the relationship between vitamin D and type 2 diabetes?

G.   What is the relationship between vitamin D and respiratory tract infections?

H.   What is the relationship between vitamin D and fibromyalgia and other diseases involving chronic pain of unknown origin?

Answers:

A. Asthma is the chronic inflammation of our airways along with a tissue hypersensitivity to invading particles and microorganisms.

B. Vitamin D promotes a reduction of symptoms. This is because it acts as an immunomodulator, decreasing tissue hypersensitivity.

C. Type 1 diabetes is characterized by the inability of insulin-producing beta cells to fulfill their role. Usually, this happens because the immune system is attacking and destroying these cells. In other cases, a genetic problem is at the root of the problem.

D. When supplemented shortly after birth, vitamin D dramatically reduces the chances of Type 1 diabetes developing.

E. In type 2 diabetes several factors come into play, with beta cells ending up being damaged by an increased in blood glucose. On the one hand, regular cells become insensitive to insulin, thus requiring beta cells to produce more and more of this hormone. On the other hand, beta cells keep running out of insulin, striving to keep up with the demand for more of this hormone. At the same time, the liver regards low insulin as a sign that glucose must be low, thus releasing its blood sugar reserves. Sugar levels rise more and more to the point of damaging various areas of the body, including the beta cells themselves — perpetuating a vicious cycle of destruction.

F. Vitamin D decreases the chances of developing type 2 diabetes. It's known that, along with vitamin K2, vitamin D increases cells' sensitivity to insulin. It's also noteworthy how the chances of developing type 2 diabetes are inversely proportional to your blood levels of vitamin D.

G. Vitamin D stimulates the immune system to attack real invaders like bacteria and viruses. Although it does not make us immune to colds and to the flu, vitamin D reduces their   incidence.

H. There seems to be a link between vitamin D deficiency and fibromyalgia and chronic pain. In addition, in the case of the muscular and skeletal pain of autoimmune or inflammatory origin, vitamin D is the treatment of choice due to its rate of remission in the order of 95% obtained by the protocol of Dr. Coimbra in his clinical practice.

Chapter 12

Vitamin D and Vitamin K2 — Risks, Benefits and Secrets

"There are risks and costs to action. But they are far less than the long range risks of comfortable inaction."

— John F. Kennedy, Politician

D o you suffer from any of the diseases mentioned in this book? In this case, it's easy to get excited about the good results being reported by the physicians involved in experimental protocols with high doses of vitamin D.

Enthusiasm is great because it motivates us to act. However, enthusiasm can't be blind, or it might endanger you or your loved ones. Throughout this book we have spoken frankly about the benefits of vitamin D and vitamin K2, revealing the secrets of the symbiotic relationship between the two, but without ever ignoring the potential risks.

Therefore, it's time to complete our exposition, wrapping up everything we have said so far. We will do this by framing the key points for each of these molecules in one of three areas:

1. Risks.
2. Benefits.
3. Secrets.

Vitamin D — the risks

The cornerstone at the heart of any possible adverse effects is only one: calcium.

When vitamin D increases it stimulates an increase in the levels of calcium in at least two ways: (1) by increasing the bowel's ability to absorb calcium from food and (2) by mobilizing the calcium present in bones, effectively promoting bone decalcification.

When calcium levels rise in our blood, the kidneys become responsible for restoring the correct values. They do this by excreting any excessive amount of calcium through the urine. This raises two problems: (1) getting high amounts of calcium flowing through your kidneys all the time increases the risk of kidney stones, and (2) if the kidney isn't working in perfect condition, excessive urination may lead to the excretion of other vital minerals together with the calcium, including potassium and magnesium.

In addition, if the kidneys fail to excrete the excessive calcium, this will lead to hypercalcemia — a condition in which calcium levels may rise to the point of impairing the correct functioning of the heart and the other organs.

Another risk of supplementing with high doses of vitamin D is related to the parathyroid gland. Excessive doses of vitamin D will suppress the production of the parathyroid hormone (PTH). This means without proper supervision, PTH levels may drop too much.

And what about vitamin K2?

Vitamin K2 — the risks

Due to the molecular similarity between vitamin K2 and vitamin K1, vitamin K2 supplementation could pose a serious risk to anyone taking anticoagulant drugs. This is because our body can convert some vitamin K1 into vitamin K2 and vice versa.

Anticoagulant therapy, like warfarin, is already dangerous, requiring close monitoring by the prescribing physician. Hence, any supplement with the potential to affect the body's ability to coagulate can never be taken without the knowledge and approval of that same specialist doctor.

Also, certain drugs, like the pill, carry a reduced but real risk of interfering with coagulation.

I don't know how healthy you are, so if you are taking any drugs on a regular basis, it would be important for you to talk to your doctor and get him to approve the addition of vitamin K2 to your protocol.

It's also worth noting the problem isn't with vitamin K2. The problem is related to the body's ability to convert vitamin K2 into vitamin K1. Since some anticoagulant drugs work by reducing vitamin K1 levels, introducing vitamin K2 could theoretically, and indirectly, increase vitamin K1 levels — hence the real risk to the user of anticoagulant drugs.

In addition to all this, it's important to note some vitamin K2 supplements also contain vitamin K1, so it's imperative to pay close attention to the labels and make them known to the medical authority in charge of your health.

And what about the risks for someone not taking anticoagulants, or other drugs that affect coagulation?

Here, a possible risk lies in the interaction between vitamin K2 and calcium. If vitamin K2 is taken without vitamin D, or in excessive amounts, it may, in theory, reduce blood calcium levels. Although this is mostly a theoretical risk, since the parathyroid gland would promptly command the bones to release their calcium into the blood, it's still a risk. One risk that can be avoided by keeping vitamin K2 dosing within the range used in the experimental protocols.

Vitamin D — the Benefits

Vitamin D in its active form is the super hormone. It seems every time a group of researchers takes vitamin D and tests it on a disease, they get positive results.

Throughout the book we have observed the effects of vitamin D on cardiovascular disease, cancer, autoimmune diseases, depression, diabetes, chronic pain and many other health issues. Even burns recover better with vitamin D.[175]

There are plenty of reasons to make vitamin D our faithful daily companion. After all, it offers not only preventive advantages, reducing by ten percentage points our probability of contracting some of the most frightening diseases, as well as real therapeutic advantages, notoriously: the treatment of autoimmune diseases.

Vitamin K2 — the Benefits

Vitamin K2 has a much humble volume of scientific research behind it — but no less impressive.

It's crucial in promoting the removal of calcium from where it shouldn't be, protecting our arteries from calcium deposits and decreasing our chances of having a heart attack. What's more, it stimulates our bones and teeth to absorb calcium, thus offering vital help in preventing, and perhaps even in resolving, osteoporosis.

But maybe its chief value is in its ability to give us an extra layer of protection against an overdose of vitamin D. Thus, vitamin K2 enhances all the therapeutic effects of vitamin D.

Vitamin D and Vitamin K2 — the secrets

In this book, my goal isn't to convince you to blindly embark on a journey of self-medication. The last thing I want is for you to get hurt while trying to follow some of the recommendations this book makes. Rather, my goal is to give you the information you need so that you can take a well-informed course of action. A course of action that by no means should exclude the support of a qualified medical doctor.

All decisions involve risks. It's up to each of us to train our faculty of discernment to **assess whether, *in our case,* the prospective benefit is sufficiently likely, and beneficial, to the point of justifying the probable risks**. In addition, it's up to us to acquire all the available information to minimize the likelihood of any risk. This is the purpose of this book: to provide you with the knowledge you need to make an informed decision.

In keeping with this goal, there are simple steps you can take to gain the benefits of vitamin D and vitamin K2 while reducing any risks. What steps are these?

Let's recap the secrets we've uncovered throughout the book.

Our primary source of vitamin D should be solar radiation. The six steps we outline to utilize the Sun as a safe source of vitamin D are the following:

1. Get out of your house because the glass windows block the ultraviolet B radiation responsible for promoting the production of vitamin D in our skin.

2. Choose the best time: between 10:00 am and 2:00 pm.

3. Don't cover your entire body with clothes. UVB radiation needs to get in direct contact with your skin.

4. Don't wear sunscreen.

5. Continue in the sun just long enough for your skin to turn pink. That means about half the time it would take for the Sun to burn your skin. Paying close attention to this reasonable time limit is especially important since the best time to be in the Sun is also the time when its radiation is most intense.

6. Avoid bathing for a few hours after sun exposure.

However, (1) if you are suffering from a disease that responds positively to vitamin D (and this would be most, if not all, illnesses), or (2) if the daily sun exposure you can enjoy is insufficient to raise your levels, then the daily intake of a vitamin D supplement is mandatory.

How can you supplement vitamin D while minimizing any risks? Let's recap the main points:

1. Start with 10,000 IU per day as this is the maximum daily dose considered safe.

2. Get your kidney function, blood calcium and urine levels, PTH and vitamin D levels tested. The vitamin D test should be the 25(OH)D — 25-hydroxycholecalciferol.

3. Understand that the goal isn't only to increase blood levels of vitamin D, but also to lower blood levels of PTH to the minimum allowed by the reference range — but not below the minimum reference value — unless under the supervision of a doctor well familiarized with high-dose vitamin D protocols.

4. Reduce calcium intake by cutting milk and its by-products from your diet, increase water consumption, avoid stress, and seek a physically active lifestyle to promote bone calcium absorption.

5. Supplement with at least vitamin K2, vitamin B2 and magnesium chloride.

6. Repeat the blood and urine tests periodically and adjust your dose of vitamin D and K2 accordingly.

7. Keep in mind that the base dose used in experimental protocols is 1,000 IU of vitamin D for every kilogram of body mass (1,000 IU per 2.20 pounds) and that this dose is further increased, or decreased, according to the laboratory work.

8. Don't forget the corresponding dose of vitamin K2: 100 mcg per 10,000 IU of vitamin D. Although in some cases, the doses of K2 used are much higher. For example, Jeff T. Bowles recommended 200 mcg of vitamin K2 MK-7 along with 1,000 mcg of vitamin K2 MK-4 for every 10,000 IU of vitamin D.

Conclusion

Have you ever heard the adage "choose your doctor, not your therapy"? That phrase is wise. In the hands of the right doctor vitamin D and vitamin K2 become powerful weapons. Also, a truly qualified physician makes use not only of this but of many other therapeutic methods, adjusting and updating them according to the progress, or regression, of the health of his patient.

Such a doctor has the power and the knowledge to ask for the right exams and the wisdom to let the test results dictate what therapeutic adjustments must be made. In this way, a properly qualified doctor is our best weapon against the degenerative processes of age and disease.

Unfortunately, nowadays many doctors are burdened under a lot of work and under the pressure exerted by the financial interests of the great pharmaceutical corporations. Because of this, finding an excellent doctor can become a journey of trial and error.

For these reasons, many people prefer to put their health in their own hands.

Such people acquire knowledge and use both books and the internet to learn about their problems and any possible solutions. When they find a therapeutic method that seems worthwhile, they invest their time and money in an even more thorough search for reliable information. If the evidence in the favor of the merit of that particular therapeutic approach mounts, a time comes when they decide to do something about it — after careful cost/benefit analysis.

That's the purpose of this book. Give you, my dear reader, the knowledge needed to distinguish the doctor who knows vitamin D and vitamin K2 from the doctor who doesn't. Moreover, it's the goal of this book to give you the power to inform your doctor about the advances in the experimental fields regarding this therapy by means of the many bibliographical references provided.

In the latter case, and especially if the reader is struggling with an autoimmune degenerative disease, or with another disease that responds positively to high doses of vitamin D, my goal is to give you hope.

Maybe vitamin D will work for you, as it has worked for 95% of Dr. Coimbra's patients and for countless other patients of similar physicians around the globe.

But what if you are in a situation where support from a qualified doctor is impossible?

There are many dangers inherent to self-medication. However, given the possibility of spending their life quadriplegic due to multiple sclerosis and the possibility of developing hypercalcemia, many people choose to try their luck, doing their best to closely follow the steps outlined by the experimental protocols, copying as closely as possible the same processes that have worked for many others before them.

This is a personal decision. In any case, if this is your decision, may this book help you in conducting your steps safely through the therapeutic process, until qualified medical help is available.

Finally, to provide you with as much help as possible, eight appendices with vital additional information were prepared. After them, you will find the section "Did you know?" Where you can learn more about my other projects.

Do you remember?

Questions:

A.   What are the risks of vitamin D?

B.   What are the risks of vitamin K2?

C.   What are the benefits of vitamin D?

D.   What are the benefits of vitamin K2?

E.   What are the secrets of Vitamin D and Vitamin K2?

Answers:

A. The fundamental risks of vitamin D supplementation involve (1) an increase in blood calcium levels, (2) bone decalcification and (3) an excessive suppression of the parathyroid gland.

B. Vitamin K2 supplementation is accompanied by the theoretical risk of (1) an excessive reduction in blood calcium levels and of it (2) being converted to vitamin K1 — which could greatly harm someone under anticoagulant drug therapy.

C. Vitamin D appears to positively influence most, if not all, degenerative processes in our body.

D. Vitamin K2 is key to a good calcium metabolism. In addition, it has the extraordinary role of providing an extra safety layer regarding the use of higher doses of vitamin D.

E. One of the secrets is the synergistic relationship between vitamin D and vitamin K2. In addition, experimental protocols and several clinical studies have uncovered many other secrets regarding the ability of vitamin D to prevent, stop and even reverse some degenerative diseases.

Other secrets involve the steps required to use the Sun, and supplementation, as a safe source of vitamin D. In the case of the Sun, these steps involve the hours you get out to get the sunlight and the care you must take so as to not take more sun than your skin can handle. In the case of supplementation, much care must be taken in avoiding calcium-rich food, maintaining a daily intake of 2.5 liters of fluids (2.64 quarts) and keeping in mind the need for physical exercise and cofactor supplementation.

The Eight Appendices
— Table of Contents

Appendix A

119 of The Foods
Highest in Vitamin D

To assist you in choosing and identifying foods rich in vitamin D, a list was prepared according to the data published in the database provided by the US Department of Agriculture, or USDA.[176]

Unless otherwise indicated, references to animal products refer to the raw state. Also, note that this list does not include fortified industrial foods nor dairy products. Therefore, if we consider the weight of 100 grams, the foods richest in vitamin D are, in order:

1. Cod liver oil, with 10,000 IU per 100 grams. Of course, no one will consume 100 grams of this oil. A realistic dose will be one tablespoon. In that case, the person will be consuming 1,360 IU of vitamin D3 for each tablespoon.

2. Mushrooms, brown, Italian, or crimini, exposed to ultraviolet light, raw: 1,276 IU. It is worth noting here, however, that the vitamin D present in these, and the remaining mushrooms, is of the D2 kind. This type of vitamin D still needs to be converted into our body, so it is not as readily available as vitamin D3.

3. Mushrooms, portabella, exposed to ultraviolet light, raw: 1135 IU.

4. Mushrooms, maitake, raw: 1123 IU.

5. Fish, halibut, Greenland, raw: 1097 IU.

6. Mushroom, white, exposed to ultraviolet light, raw: 1046 IU.

7. Fish, mackerel, salted: 1006 IU.

8. Fish, carp, raw: 988 IU.

9. Fish, eel, mixed species, raw: 932 IU.

10. Salmon, sockeye, canned, drained solids, without skin and bones: 859 IU.

11. Fish, salmon, sockeye, canned, drained solids: 841 IU.

12. Salmon, sockeye, canned, total can contents: 761 IU.

13. Fish, trout, rainbow, farmed, cooked, dry heat: 759 IU.

14. Fish, salmon, chinook, smoked: 685 IU.

15. Fish, salmon, sockeye, cooked, dry heat: 670 IU.

16. Fish, swordfish, cooked, dry heat: 666 IU.

17. Fish, mackerel, Atlantic, raw: 643 IU.

18. Fish, sturgeon, mixed species, smoked: 642 IU.

19. Fish, trout, rainbow, farmed, raw: 635 IU.

20. Fish, salmon, pink, canned, drained solids: 580 IU.

21. Fish, salmon, sockeye, raw: 563 IU.

22. Fish, Salmon, pink, canned, drained solids, without skin and bones: 563 IU.

23. Fish, swordfish, raw: 558 IU.

24. Fish, salmon, pink, canned, total can contents: 547 IU.

25. Fish, cisco, smoked: 530 IU.

26. Fish, salmon, Atlantic, farmed, cooked, dry heat: 526 IU.

27. Mushrooms, portabella, exposed to ultraviolet light, grilled: 524 IU.

28. Fish, salmon, pink, cooked, dry heat: 522 IU.

29. Fish, sturgeon, mixed species, cooked, dry heat: 515 IU.

30. Fish, whitefish, mixed species, smoked: 512 IU.

31. Fish, catfish, channel, wild, raw: 500 IU.

32. Fish, roe, mixed species, raw: 484 IU.

33. Fish, whitefish, mixed species, raw: 478 IU.

34. Fish, mackerel, Pacific and jack, mixed species, cooked, dry heat: 457 IU.

35. Fish, salmon, coho, wild, cooked, dry heat: 451 IU.

36. Fish, salmon, Atlantic, farmed, raw: 441 IU.

37. Fish, pompano, Florida, raw: 439 IU.

38. Fish, salmon, pink, raw: 435 IU.

39. Egg, yolk, dried: 417 IU.

40. Fish, sturgeon, mixed species, raw: 412 IU.

41. Fish, snapper, mixed species, raw: 408 IU.

42. Fish, salmon, chum, canned, drained solids with bone: 386 IU.

43. Fish, mackerel, Pacific and jack, mixed species, raw: 366 IU.

44. Fish, salmon, coho, wild, raw: 361 IU.

45. Fish oil, sardine: 332 IU.

46. Egg, whole, dried: 331 IU.

47. Egg Mix, USDA Commodity: 296 IU.

48. Fish, mackerel, jack, canned, drained solids: 292 IU.

49. Fish, mackerel, Spanish, raw: 292 IU.

50. Fish, tuna, light, canned in oil, drained solids: 269 IU.

51. Egg, yolk, raw, frozen, pasteurized: 238 IU.

52. Fish, halibut, Atlantic and Pacific, cooked, dry heat: 231 IU.

53. Fish, tuna, fresh, bluefin, raw: 227 IU.

54. Fish, sea bass, mixed species, raw: 226 IU.

55. Egg, yolk, raw, fresh: 218 IU.

56. Fish, herring, Atlantic, cooked, dry heat: 214 IU.

57. Mushrooms, Chanterelle, raw: 212 IU.

58. Mushrooms, morel, raw: 206 IU.

59. Fish, sardine, Atlantic, canned in oil, drained solids with bone: 193 IU.

60. Fish, sardine, Pacific, canned in tomato sauce, drained solids with bone: 193 IU.

61. Fat, chicken: 191 IU.

62. Fat, duck: 191 IU.

63. Fat, turkey: 191 IU.

64. Fish, halibut, Atlantic and Pacific, raw: 190 IU.

65. Fish, shad, American, raw: 190 IU.

66. Fish, shad, American, raw: 190 IU.

67. Fish, rockfish, Pacific, mixed species, cooked, dry heat: 183 IU.

68. Fish, herring, Atlantic, raw: 167 IU.

69. Fish, cod, Atlantic, dried and salted: 161 IU.

70. Fish, trout, mixed species, raw: 155 IU.

71. Mushrooms, shiitake, dried: 154 IU.

72. Fish, rockfish, Pacific, mixed species, raw: 151 IU.

73. Fish, tilapia, cooked, dry heat: 150 IU.

74. Fish, flatfish (flounder and sole species), cooked, dry heat: 139 IU.

75. Chicken, broilers or fryers, separable fat, raw: 130 IU.

76. Egg, yolk, raw, frozen, salted, pasteurized: 126 IU.

77. Seaweed, Canadian Cultivated EMI–TSUNOMATA, dry: 126 IU.

78. Fish, tilapia, raw: 124 IU.

79. Egg, yolk, raw, frozen, sugared, pasteurized: 123 IU.

80. Pork, fresh, backfat, raw: 122 IU.

81. Fish, perch, mixed species, raw: 118 IU.

82. Fish, caviar, black and red, granular: 117 IU.

83. Fish, flatfish (flounder and sole species), raw: 113 IU.

84. Fish, herring, Atlantic, pickled: 113 IU.

85. Cheese, fresh, queso fresco: 110 IU.

86. Egg, whole, raw, frozen, pasteurized: 105 IU.

87. Pork, fresh, spareribs, separable lean and fat, cooked, braised: 104 IU.

88. Lard: 102 IU.

89. Animal fat, bacon grease: 101 IU.

90. Meat drippings (lard, beef tallow, mutton tallow): 100 IU.

91. Fish, pike, northern, raw: 99 IU.

92. Pork, cured, ham, extra lean (approximately 4% fat), canned, unheated: 93 IU.

93. Pork, fresh, spareribs, separable lean and fat, raw: 91 IU.

94. Egg, whole, cooked, fried: 88 IU.

95. Pork, fresh, spareribs, separable lean and fat, cooked, roasted: 88 IU.

96. Egg, whole, cooked, hard-boiled: 87 IU.

97. Fish, herring, Atlantic, kippered: 86 IU.

98. Egg, whole, raw, fresh: 82 IU.

99. Egg, whole, cooked, poached: 82 IU.

100. Fish, tuna, yellowfin, fresh, cooked, dry heat: 82 IU.

101. Fish, tuna, white, canned in water, drained solids: 80 IU.

102. Turkey and pork sausage, fresh, bulk, patty or link, cooked: 79 IU.

103. Pork, cured, ham, separable fat, boneless, heated: 75 IU.

104. Cheese, dry white, queso seco: 73 IU.

105. Fish, whiting, mixed species, cooked, dry heat: 73 IU.

106. Egg, whole, cooked, scrambled: 72 IU.

107. Pork, fresh, separable fat, cooked: 72 IU.

108. Pork, fresh, loin, country-style ribs, separable lean and fat, bone-in, cooked, roasted: 72 IU.

109. Eggs, scrambled, frozen mixture: 72 IU.
110. Pork, fresh, shoulder, whole, separable lean and fat, raw: 70 IU.
111. Egg, whole, cooked, omelet: 69 IU.
112. Egg, duck, whole, fresh, raw: 69 IU.
113. Pork, fresh, separable fat, raw: 69 IU.
114. Fish, anchovy, European, canned in oil, drained solids: 69 IU.
115. Fish, tuna, fresh, yellowfin, raw: 69 IU.
116. Veal, loin, separable lean and fat, raw: 69 IU.
117. Egg, goose, whole, fresh, raw: 66 IU.
118. Egg substitute, liquid or frozen, fat-free: 66 IU.
119. Cream, fluid, heavy whipping: 63

It is worth noting that if you eat fish you **should not eat the fishbones** because they are rich in calcium. Now you may be thinking, "Why would I eat the fishbones?" Well, the truth is that when we eat canned sardines, for example, we can end up eating some of the fishbones even without noticing it. Hence the additional warning.

Appendix B

240 Foods Listed by The USDA Containing 1,0 Or More Micrograms of Vitamin K2 per 100 Grams

Now, to assist you in the identification of vitamin K2 rich foods a list was prepared, based mainly on data published in the database provided by the United States Department of Agriculture, or USDA. This list includes some relevant food products of industrial origin. Also, regarding the USDA, even though the data published by this entity allow us to access hundreds of nutritional parameters from thousands of foods, they only list the values for vitamin K1 and vitamin K2 MK-4. No reference to vitamin K2 MK-7! This helps us to fully grasp how relatively unexplored the field of vitamin K2 research is.

In addition, many other websites I've consulted, providing supposed lists of vitamin K2 rich foods, end up mixing vitamin K1 with K2 and do not reveal their sources. This makes these lists effectively useless. As such, for the vitamin K2 MK-7 values present in natto, this book uses the results published in a Japanese study by the *Central Research Institute*.[177]

According to reliable sources, and if we consider the weight of 100 grams, the foods containing 1 or more micrograms of vitamin K2, are, in order:

1. Natto (fermented soybeans): Between 775 mcg and 1765 mcg. (Vitamin K2 MK-7)

2. Pepperoni, beef and pork, sliced: 41.7 mcg.

3. Sausage, turkey, breakfast links, mild, raw: 36.6 mcg.

4. Chicken, broilers or fryers, drumstick, rotisserie, original seasoning, meat only, cooked: 35.7 mcg.

5. Frankfurter, meat and poultry, cooked, grilled: 35.6 mcg.

6. Chicken, broilers or fryers, rotisserie, original seasoning, drumstick, meat and skin, cooked: 33.2 mcg.

7. Frankfurter, turkey: 31.2 mcg.

8. Frankfurter, meat and poultry, unheated: 28.6 mcg.

9. Meatballs, frozen, Italian style: 28.1 mcg.

10. Salami, cooked, beef and pork: 28.0 mcg.

11. Chicken, broilers or fryers, rotisserie, original seasoning, wing, meat only, cooked: 27.5 mcg.

12. Chicken, broilers or fryers, rotisserie, original seasoning, back, meat only, cooked: 25.6 mcg.

13. Chicken, broilers or fryers, rotisserie, original seasoning, wing, meat and skin, cooked: 25.3 mcg.

14. Frankfurter, chicken: 25.1 mcg.

15. Chicken, broilers or fryers, rotisserie, original seasoning, back, meat and skin, cooked: 24.3 mcg.

16. Chicken, broilers or fryers, rotisserie, original seasoning, thigh, meat only, cooked: 24.0 mcg.

17. Chicken, broilers or fryers, wing, meat and skin, raw: 23.7 mcg.

18. Chicken, broilers or fryers, rotisserie, original seasoning, thigh, meat and skin, cooked: 23.5 mcg.

19. Pork sausage, link/patty, fully cooked, microwaved: 22.5 mcg.

20. Butter, whipped, with salt: 20.9 mcg.

21. Chicken, broilers or fryers, rotisserie, original seasoning, skin only, cooked: 20.9 mcg.

22. Kielbasa, fully cooked, grilled: 20.1 mcg.

23. Chicken, skin (drumsticks and thighs), with added solution, cooked, roasted: 19.6 mcg.

24. Chicken, skin (drumsticks and thighs), with added solution, raw: 19.5 mcg.

25. Babyfood, meat, turkey, strained: 18.7 mcg.

26. Babyfood, meat, turkey, junior: 18.7 mcg.

27. Pork sausage, link/patty, fully cooked, unheated: 18.7 mcg.

28. Pork sausage, link/patty, unprepared: 18.3 mcg.

29. Kielbasa, fully cooked, unheated: 15.7 mcg.

30. Chicken, broilers or fryers, rotisserie, original seasoning, breast, meat and skin, cooked: 15.5 mcg.

31. Cheese, pasteurized process, American, fortified with vitamin D: 14.1 mcg.

32. Sausage, smoked link sausage, pork: 13.7 mcg.

33. Chicken, dark meat, drumstick, meat and skin, with added solution, cooked, roasted: 13.5 mcg.

34. Chicken, dark meat, thigh, meat and skin, with added solution, cooked, roasted: 13.1 mcg.

35. Chicken, dark meat, drumstick, meat only, with added solution, cooked, roasted: 12.7 mcg.

36. DENNY'S, chicken nuggets, star-shaped, from kid's menu: 12.6 mcg.

37. Chicken, dark meat, thigh, meat and skin, with added solution, raw: 12.0 mcg.

38. Chicken, dark meat, thigh, meat only, with added solution, cooked, roasted: 11.6 mcg.

39. Chicken, broiler or fryers, breast, skinless, boneless, meat only, cooked, grilled: 11.1 mcg.

40. Corn dogs, frozen, prepared: 11.1 mcg.

41. Chicken, dark meat, drumstick, meat and skin, with added solution, raw: 11.0 mcg.

42. Chicken, broilers or fryers, breast, skinless, boneless, meat only, with added solution, raw: 10.5 mcg.

43. Pork, cured, feet, pickled: 10.4 mcg.

44. KFC, Crispy Chicken Strips: 10.3 mcg.

45. Chicken pot pie, frozen entree, prepared: 9.9 mcg.

46. Pork, cured, ham with natural juices, rump, bone-in, separable lean only, heated, roasted: 9.6 mcg.

47. Chicken, dark meat, drumstick, meat only, with added solution, raw: 9.5 mcg.

48. Cheese, neufchatel: 9.3 mcg.

49. Cheese food, pasteurized process, American, without added vitamin D: 8.9 mcg.

50. Cheese, cream: 8.7 mcg.

51. Cheese, cheddar, sharp, sliced: 8.6 mcg.

52. Cheese, cheddar (Includes foods for USDA's Food Distribution Program): 8.6 mcg.

53. Pork, cured, ham with natural juices, rump, bone-in, separable lean and fat, heated, roasted: 8.6 mcg.

54. Chicken, dark meat, thigh, meat only, with added solution, raw: 8.5 mcg.

55. Chicken, broiler or fryers, breast, skinless, boneless, meat only, raw: 8.4 mcg.

56. APPLEBEE'S, chicken tenders, from kids' menu: 8.2 mcg.

57. Restaurant, Chinese, general tso's chicken: 7.2 mcg.

58. Cheese, parmesan, grated: 7.1 mcg.

59. Pork, cured, ham with natural juices, shank, bone-in, separable lean only, heated, roasted: 7.1 mcg.

60. KFC, Popcorn Chicken: 7.1 mcg.

61. Restaurant, family style, chicken fingers, from kid's menu: 6.9 mcg.

62. Chicken tenders, breaded, frozen, prepared: 6.6 mcg.

63. T.G.I. FRIDAY'S, chicken fingers, from kids' menu: 6.4 mcg.

64. Cheese, swiss: 6.3 mcg.

65. Bologna, beef: 6.3 mcg.

66. Pork, cured, ham with natural juices, shank, bone-in, separable lean and fat, heated, roasted: 6.2 mcg.

67. Pork, cured, ham and water product, rump, bone-in, separable lean only, heated, roasted: 6.1 mcg.

68. Pork, pickled pork hocks: 6.0 mcg.

69. Cream, sour, cultured: 6.0 mcg.

70. Cheese, dry white, queso seco: 5.9 mcg.

71. CRACKER BARREL, chicken tenderloin platter, fried, from kid's menu: 5.9 mcg.

72. Cheese, white, queso blanco: 5.8 mcg.

73. Pork, cured, ham — water added, shank, bone-in, separable lean only, heated, roasted: 5.6 mcg.

74. Pork, cured, ham with natural juices, slice, bone-in, separable lean only, heated, pan-broil: 5.5 mcg.

75. Cheese, cream, low fat: 5.4 mcg.

76. Babyfood, meat, lamb, strained: 5.3 mcg.

77. Pork, cured, ham and water product, rump, bone-in, separable lean and fat, heated, roasted: 5.2 mcg.

78. Pork, cured, ham with natural juices, slice, bone-in, separable lean and fat, heated, pan-broil: 5.1 mcg.

79. Cheese product, pasteurized process, American, vitamin D fortified: 5.0 mcg.

80. Mollusks, oyster, eastern, wild, cooked, moist heat: 5.0 mcg.

81. Canadian bacon, cooked, pan-fried: 4.9 mcg.

82. Restaurant, Latino, chicken and rice, entree, prepared: 4.8 mcg.

83. Pork, cured, ham and water product, shank, bone-in, separable lean only, heated, roasted: 4.8 mcg.

84. Pork, cured, ham — water added, shank, bone-in, separable lean and fat, heated, roasted: 4.5 mcg.

85. Pork, cured, ham and water product, slice, boneless, separable lean and fat, heated, pan-broil: 4.5 mcg.

86. Pie crust, refrigerated, regular, baked: 4.5 mcg.

87. Pork, cured, ham and water product, slice, boneless, separable lean only, heated, pan-broil: 4.5 mcg.

88. Ham, sliced, pre-packaged, deli meat (96%fat free, water added): 4.4 mcg.

89. Pork, cured, ham and water product, whole, boneless, separable lean only, unheated: 4.3 mcg.

90. Pork, cured, ham and water product, whole, boneless, separable lean and fat, unheated: 4.3 mcg.

91. Dulce de Leche: 4.2 mcg.

92. Cheese, mozzarella, low moisture, part-skim, shredded: 4.1 mcg.

93. Pork, cured, ham — water added, whole, boneless, separable lean only, heated, roasted: 4.1 mcg.

94. Cheese, mozzarella, low moisture, part-skim: 4.1 mcg.

95. Babyfood, dinner, broccoli and chicken, junior: 4.1 mcg.

96. Pie crust, refrigerated, regular, unbaked: 4.0 mcg.

97. Pork, cured, ham — water added, slice, boneless, separable lean only, heated, pan-broil: 4.0 mcg.

98. Pork, cured, ham — water added, whole, boneless, separable lean and fat, heated, roasted: 4.0 mcg.

99. Pork, cured, ham and water product, whole, boneless, separable lean and fat, heated, roasted: 4.0 mcg.

100. DIGIORNO Pizza, pepperoni topping, thin crispy crust, frozen, baked: 4.0 mcg.

101. Pork, cured, ham — water added, slice, boneless, separable lean and fat, heated, pan-broil: 4.0 mcg.

102. Pork, cured, ham and water product, whole, boneless, separable lean only, heated, roasted: 4.0 mcg.

103. Mollusks, oyster, eastern, wild, cooked, dry heat: 3.9 mcg.

104. Pork, cured, ham with natural juices, spiral slice, meat only, boneless, separable lean only, heated, roasted: 3.6 mcg.

105. Cheese, fresh, queso fresco: 3.6 mcg.

106. DENNY'S, top sirloin steak: 3.5 mcg.

107. Pork, cured, ham and water product, shank, bone-in, separable lean and fat, heated, roasted: 3.5 mcg.

108. Pork, cured, ham — water added, whole, boneless, separable lean only, unheated: 3.5 mcg.

109. Canadian bacon, unprepared: 3.5 mcg.

110. CRACKER BARREL, grilled sirloin steak: 3.5 mcg.

111. Pork, cured, ham with natural juices, spiral slice, boneless, separable lean and fat, heated, roasted: 3.5 mcg.

112. DIGIORNO Pizza, supreme topping, thin crispy crust, frozen, baked: 3.4 mcg.

113. Pork, cured, ham — water added, slice, bone-in, separable lean only, heated, pan-broil: 3.4 mcg.

114. Soup, hot and sour, Chinese restaurant: 3.4 mcg.

115. Pork, cured, ham — water added, whole, boneless, separable lean and fat, unheated: 3.4 mcg.

116. Pork, cured, ham with natural juices, whole, boneless, separable lean only, unheated: 3.3 mcg.

117. Restaurant, Chinese, egg rolls, assorted: 3.3 mcg.

118. Pork, cured, ham with natural juices, slice, boneless, separable lean and fat, heated, pan-broil: 3.2 mcg.

119. Restaurant, Italian, lasagna with meat: 3.2 mcg.

120. OLIVE GARDEN, lasagna classico: 3.2 mcg.

121. DIGIORNO Pizza, cheese topping, cheese stuffed crust, frozen, baked: 3.2 mcg.

122. Pork, cured, ham and water product, slice, bone-in, separable lean only, heated, pan-broil: 3.2 mcg.

123. Pork, cured, ham with natural juices, whole, boneless, separable lean and fat, unheated: 3.2 mcg.

124. Beef, chuck, shoulder clod, top blade, steak, separable lean and fat, trimmed to 0" fat, choice, raw: 3.2 mcg.

125. Beef, chuck, shoulder clod, top blade, steak, separable lean and fat, trimmed to 0" fat, all grades, raw: 3.2 mcg.

126. Pork, cured, ham with natural juices, slice, boneless, separable lean only, heated, pan-broil: 3.2 mcg.

127. Gravy, HEINZ Home Style, classic chicken: 3.1 mcg.

128. Beef, chuck, shoulder clod, top blade, steak, separable lean and fat, trimmed to 0" fat, choice, cooked, grilled: 3.1 mcg.

129. Pork, cured, ham — water added, slice, bone-in, separable lean and fat, heated, pan-broil: 3.1 mcg.

130. Beef, chuck, shoulder clod, top blade, steak, separable lean and fat, trimmed to 0" fat, select, cooked, grilled: 3.1 mcg.

131. Beef, chuck, shoulder clod, top blade, steak, separable lean and fat, trimmed to 0" fat, all grades, cooked, grilled: 3.1 mcg.

132. Beef, chuck, shoulder clod, top blade, steak, separable lean and fat, trimmed to 0" fat, select, raw: 3.1 mcg.

133. DIGIORNO Pizza, supreme topping, rising crust, frozen, baked: 3.0 mcg.

134. Pork, cured, ham and water product, slice, bone-in, separable lean and fat, heated, pan-broil: 2.9 mcg.

135. McDONALD's, Southern Style Chicken Biscuit: 2.9 mcg.

136. Restaurant, Latino, tamale, pork: 2.9 mcg.

137. Fast foods, biscuit, with crispy chicken fillet: 2.9 mcg.

138. Restaurant, Latino, pupusas con queso (pupusas, cheese): 2.9 mcg.

139. Restaurant, Latino, pupusas del cerdo (pupusas, pork): 2.9 mcg.

140. DIGIORNO Pizza, pepperoni topping, cheese stuffed crust, frozen, baked: 2.8 mcg.

141. PIZZA HUT 14" Cheese Pizza, THIN 'N CRISPY Crust: 2.8 mcg.

142. Gravy, chicken, canned or bottled, ready-to-serve: 2.7 mcg.

143. DIGIORNO Pizza, pepperoni topping, rising crust, frozen, baked: 2.7 mcg.

144. Tamales, masa and pork filling (Hopi): 2.7 mcg.

145. Restaurant, Latino, empanadas, beef, prepared: 2.6 mcg.

146. Restaurant, Chinese, lemon chicken: 2.6 mcg.

147. Pork, cured, ham — water added, rump, bone-in, separable lean only, heated, roasted: 2.5 mcg.

148. Mollusks, oyster, eastern, wild, raw: 2.5 mcg.

149. PIZZA HUT 14" Pepperoni Pizza, Hand-Tossed Crust: 2.5 mcg.

150. Pork, cured, ham with natural juices, whole, boneless, separable lean and fat, heated, roasted: 2.4 mcg.

151. Restaurant, Chinese, sweet and sour chicken: 2.4 mcg.

152. Pork, cured, ham with natural juices, whole, boneless, separable lean only, heated, roasted: 2.4 mcg.

153. Restaurant, Latino, tripe soup: 2.4 mcg.

154. Restaurant, family style, fried mozzarella sticks: 2.3 mcg.

155. APPLEBEE'S, mozzarella sticks: 2.3 mcg.

156. Pork, cured, ham — water added, rump, bone-in, separable lean and fat, heated, roasted: 2.3 mcg.

157. Restaurant, Chinese, shrimp and vegetables: 2.3 mcg.

158. Beef Pot Pie, frozen entree, prepared: 2.2 mcg.

159. Rolls, dinner, sweet: 2.2 mcg.

160. Restaurant, Chinese, kung pao chicken: 2.2 mcg.

161. DENNY'S, mozzarella cheese sticks: 2.1 mcg.

162. Restaurant, Latino, bunuelos (fried yeast bread): 2.1 mcg.

163. Rice bowl with chicken, frozen entree, prepared (includes fried, teriyaki, and sweet and sour varieties): 2.1 mcg.

164. PIZZA HUT 14" Pepperoni Pizza, Pan Crust: 2.1 mcg.

165. Pie crust, standard-type, frozen, ready-to-bake, enriched, baked: 2.0 mcg.

166. Beef, round, outside round, bottom round, steak, separable lean and fat, trimmed to 0" fat, select, cooked, grilled: 2.0 mcg.

167. Pork, cured, ham, slice, bone-in, separable lean only, heated, pan-broil: 2.0 mcg.

168. PIZZA HUT 14" Super Supreme Pizza, Hand-Tossed Crust: 2.0 mcg.

169. Restaurant, Chinese, sweet and sour pork: 2.0 mcg.

170. Fast Food, Pizza Chain, 14" pizza, meat and vegetable topping, regular crust: 2.0 mcg.

171. Restaurant, Chinese, beef and vegetables: 2.0 mcg.

172. Oil, flaxseed, contains added sliced flaxseed: 2.0 mcg.

173. Beef, chuck, shoulder clod, shoulder top and center steaks, separable lean and fat, trimmed to 0" fat, select, cooked, grilled: 1.9 mcg.

174. Beef, round, outside round, bottom round, steak, separable lean and fat, trimmed to 0" fat, choice, cooked, grilled: 1.9 mcg.

175. DIGIORNO Pizza, cheese topping, thin crispy crust, frozen, baked: 1.9 mcg.

176. Beef, round, outside round, bottom round, steak, separable lean and fat, trimmed to 0" fat, all grades, cooked, grilled: 1.9 mcg.

177. Pie crust, standard-type, frozen, ready-to-bake, enriched: 1.8 mcg.

178. Pork, cured, ham, slice, bone-in, separable lean and fat, heated, pan-broil: 1.8 mcg.

179. Beef, round, knuckle, tip side, steak, separable lean and fat, trimmed to 0" fat, all grades, cooked, grilled: 1.8 mcg.

180. HOT POCKETS Ham 'N Cheese Stuffed Sandwich, frozen: 1.8 mcg.

181. Beef, round, knuckle, tip side, steak, separable lean and fat, trimmed to 0" fat, choice, cooked, grilled: 1.8 mcg.

182. Beef, chuck, shoulder clod, shoulder top and center steaks, separable lean and fat, trimmed to 0" fat, all grades, cooked, grilled: 1.8 mcg.

183. Beef, chuck, shoulder clod, shoulder top and center steaks, separable lean and fat, trimmed to 0" fat, choice, cooked, grilled: 1.8 mcg.

184. Pork, cured, ham, rump, bone-in, separable lean only, heated, roasted: 1.7 mcg.

185. Beef, round, outside round, bottom round, steak, separable lean and fat, trimmed to 0" fat, choice, raw: 1.7 mcg.

186. Beef, round, knuckle, tip side, steak, separable lean and fat, trimmed to 0" fat, select, cooked, grilled: 1.7 mcg.

187. Gravy, CAMPBELL'S, chicken: 1.7 mcg.

188. Beef, round, outside round, bottom round, steak, separable lean and fat, trimmed to 0" fat, all grades, raw: 1.7 mcg.

189. Margarine-like, margarine-butter blend, soybean oil and butter: 1.7 mcg.

190. Pork, cured, ham, slice, bone-in, separable lean only, unheated: 1.6 mcg.

191. Beef, round, knuckle, tip center, steak, separable lean and fat, trimmed to 0" fat, choice, cooked, grilled: 1.6 mcg.

192. HOT POCKETS, meatballs & mozzarella stuffed sandwich, frozen: 1.6 mcg.

193. Beef, round, knuckle, tip center, steak, separable lean and fat, trimmed to 0" fat, all grades, cooked, grilled: 1.6 mcg.

194. Pork, cured, ham, shank, bone-in, separable lean only, heated, roasted: 1.6 mcg.

195. Beef, round, knuckle, tip center, steak, separable lean and fat, trimmed to 0" fat, choice, raw: 1.5 mcg.

196. Beef, round, knuckle, tip center, steak, separable lean and fat, trimmed to 0" fat, all grades, raw: 1.5 mcg.

197. Beef, chuck, shoulder clod, shoulder tender, medallion, separable lean and fat, trimmed to 0" fat, choice, raw: 1.5 mcg.

198. Pulled pork in barbecue sauce: 1.5 mcg.

199. Beef, chuck, shoulder clod, shoulder top and center steaks, separable lean and fat, trimmed to 0" fat, choice, raw: 1.5 mcg.

200. Pork, cured, ham, rump, bone-in, separable lean and fat, heated, roasted: 1.5 mcg.

201. Beef, round, knuckle, tip center, steak, separable lean and fat, trimmed to 0" fat, select, cooked, grilled: 1.5 mcg.

202. Beef, round, knuckle, tip center, steak, separable lean and fat, trimmed to 0" fat, select, raw: 1.5 mcg.

203. Babyfood, meat, veal, strained: 1.5 mcg.

204. Beef, chuck, shoulder clod, shoulder top and center steaks, separable lean and fat, trimmed to 0" fat, select, raw: 1.5 mcg.

205. Beef, chuck, shoulder clod, shoulder tender, medallion, separable lean and fat, trimmed to 0" fat, select, raw: 1.5 mcg.

206. Beef, chuck, shoulder clod, shoulder top and center steaks, separable lean and fat, trimmed to 0" fat, all grades, raw: 1.5 mcg.

207. Beef, chuck, shoulder clod, shoulder tender, medallion, separable lean and fat, trimmed to 0" fat, all grades, raw: 1.5 mcg.

208. LEAN POCKETS, Ham N Cheddar: 1.5 mcg.

209. DIGIORNO Pizza, cheese topping, rising crust, frozen, baked: 1.4 mcg.

210. Pork, cured, ham, slice, bone-in, separable lean and fat, unheated: 1.4 mcg.

211. Lasagna with meat sauce, frozen, prepared: 1.4 mcg.

212. Pork, cured, ham, shank, bone-in, separable lean and fat, heated, roasted: 1.4 mcg.

213. Beef, round, outside round, bottom round, steak, separable lean and fat, trimmed to 0" fat, select, raw: 1.4 mcg.

214. Pork, cured, ham, rump, bone-in, separable lean only, unheated: 1.4 mcg.

215. Taquitos, frozen, beef and cheese, oven-heated: 1.4 mcg.

216. Beef, chuck, shoulder clod, shoulder tender, medallion, separable lean and fat, trimmed to 0" fat, select, cooked, grilled: 1.3 mcg.

217. Pork, cured, ham, shank, bone-in, separable lean only, unheated: 1.3 mcg.

218. Beef, chuck, shoulder clod, shoulder tender, medallion, separable lean and fat, trimmed to 0" fat, choice, cooked, grilled: 1.3 mcg.

219. PIZZA HUT 14" Cheese Pizza, Hand-Tossed Crust: 1.3 mcg.

220. Beef, chuck, shoulder clod, shoulder tender, medallion, separable lean and fat, trimmed to 0" fat, all grades, cooked, grilled: 1.3 mcg.

221. Beef, round, knuckle, tip side, steak, separable lean and fat, trimmed to 0" fat, select, raw: 1.2 mcg.

222. Pork, cured, ham, shank, bone-in, separable lean and fat, unheated: 1.2 mcg.

223. Pie crust, deep dish, frozen, unbaked, made with enriched flour: 1.2 mcg.

224. Restaurant, Chinese, chicken chow mein: 1.2 mcg.

225. Lasagna with meat & sauce, frozen entree: 1.2 mcg.

226. Beef, round, knuckle, tip side, steak, separable lean and fat, trimmed to 0" fat, all grades, raw: 1.2 mcg.

227. Beef, round, knuckle, tip side, steak, separable lean and fat, trimmed to 0" fat, choice, raw: 1.2 mcg.

228. Caribou, hind quarter, meat, cooked (Alaska Native): 1.2 mcg.

229. Pork, cured, ham, rump, bone-in, separable lean and fat, unheated: 1.2 mcg.

230. Lean Pockets, Meatballs & Mozzarella: 1.1 mcg.

231. Fast foods, breadstick, soft, prepared with garlic and parmesan cheese: 1.1 mcg.

232. PIZZA HUT 14" Cheese Pizza, Pan Crust: 1.1 mcg.

233. Quinoa, uncooked: 1.1 mcg.

234. CRACKER BARREL, macaroni n' cheese plate, from kid's menu: 1.1 mcg.

235. PIZZA HUT, breadstick, parmesan garlic: 1.1 mcg.

236. Milk, whole, 3.25% milkfat, without added vitamin A and vitamin D: 1.0 mcg.

237. Pie crust, deep dish, frozen, baked, made with enriched flour: 1.0 mcg.

238. Restaurant, Latino, arepa (unleavened cornmeal bread): 1.0 mcg.

239. ON THE BORDER, refried beans: 1.0 mcg.

240. Milk, whole, 3.25% milkfat, with added vitamin D: 1.0 mcg.

Note that many of these foods — like cheese and butter — **are contraindicated in a high-dose vitamin D protocol because of their elevated calcium content.**

Appendix C

Foods to Avoid During High-Dose Vitamin D Therapy And Foods to Eat in Moderation

For all the reasons already presented, calcium is a mineral that needs to be kept under surveillance while on the experimental protocols. As such, and as directed by Dr. Coimbra, milk and its by-products are contraindicated because of their high calcium content. Other calcium-rich foods, however, may go unnoticed, such as wheat bread or tofu prepared with calcium sulfate.

This list is designed to help you in two ways:

- First, it helps you understand the amount of calcium present in various foods, so you can better understand what other foods have calcium levels similar to dairy products.

- Second, this list may help if you if are finding it difficult to keep your calcium levels within the recommended range.

When you begin supplementing with high-dose vitamin D, you should only worry about cutting dairy products and reducing the consumption of wheat bread — as well as cutting out cereals and other foods <u>fortified</u> with calcium.

However, if your blood and urine tests reveal that your calcium levels are getting higher, this indicates you need to further reduce your calcium intake. If this is the case, use this list to check if you are ingesting any of the non-dairy foods referenced at the top and try to reduce the amount you are consuming. To facilitate your search, all non-dairy foods are highlighted.

On the other hand, if your calcium levels are dropping too much, getting close to the minimum recommended values, this may be a sign that you need to introduce some non-dairy calcium-containing foods in your diet, throughout the week. You can start by introducing into your diet foods from the nearer bottom of the list. Subsequently, adjust what non-dairy calcium-containing foods you will allow in your diet according to the results of future blood work.

This list was prepared using two databases, the USDA[178] database and the database provided by the Portuguese National Health Service.[179, 180] It presents information on foods with more than 100 milligrams of calcium per 100 grams. The original sources referenced can be consulted directly by the reader for even more complete information.

For every 100 grams of food, the amount of calcium in milligrams is:

1. **Tofu, koyadofu, prepared with calcium sulfate:** 2134 mg.

2. **Parmesan cheese:** 1300 mg.

3. **Milk, dry, nonfat, regular, without added vitamin A and vitamin D:** 1270 mg.

4. **Ground cinnamon:** 1230 mg. Note, however, that this value is for 100 grams of cinnamon. One teaspoon, equivalent to 2.6 grams of cinnamon, contains about 31 milligrams of calcium.

5. **Milk, buttermilk, dried:** 1184 mg.

6. **Milk, semi-skimmed powdered milk:** 1150 mg.

7. **Cheese, Emmental:** 1080 mg.

8. **Cheese pasteurized, American, fortified with vitamin D:** 1045 mg.

9. **Milk, full fat powdered milk:** 920 mg.

10. **Cheese, swiss:** 890 mg.

11. **Flemish cheese 30% fat:** 850 mg.

12. **Parmesan cheese topping, fat-free:** 800 mg.

13. **Flemish cheese 45% fat:** 800 mg.

14. **Whey, sweet, dried:** 796 mg.

15. **Cheese, pasteurized process, swiss:** 772 mg.

16. **Cheese, Roquefort:** 770 mg.

17. **Cheese, provolone:** 756 mg.

18. **Molten cheese 40% fat:** 750 mg.
19. **Cheese, muenster:** 717 mg.
20. **Cheese, cheddar:** 710 mg.
21. **Cheese, mozzarella, low moisture, part-skim:** 697 mg.
22. <u>**Bread, white wheat:**</u> 684 mg.
23. <u>**Tofu, raw, firm, prepared with calcium sulfate:**</u> 683 mg.
24. **Cheese, mexican, queso chihuahua:** 651 mg.
25. **Cheese spread, pasteurized process, American:** 562 mg.
26. **Cheese, blue:** 528 mg.
27. **Cheese, mozzarella, whole milk:** 505 mg.
28. <u>**Wheat and rice flakes enriched with vitamins, calcium and iron:**</u> 500 mg.
29. **Cheese, feta:** 493 mg.
30. <u>**Vegetable sour cream 58% fat, with calcium:**</u> 480 mg.
31. <u>**Pancakes, buckwheat, dry mix, incomplete:**</u> 476 mg.
32. <u>**Canned sardine, semi-skimmed, preserved in olive oil (drained):**</u> 470 mg.
33. **13% protein curd:** 470 mg.
34. <u>**Chocolate powder with high-fat content:**</u> 420 mg.
35. **Cheese, Camembert:** 388 mg.
36. <u>**Cornmeal, white, self-rising, degermed, enriched:**</u> 350 mg.
37. <u>**Carob flour:**</u> 350 mg.
38. <u>**Nuts, almond butter, plain, with salt added:**</u> 347 mg.
39. **Condensed milk, cow:** 340 mg.
40. <u>**Egg substitute, powder:**</u> 326 mg.
41. <u>**Ham and pineapple pizza — filling:**</u> 320 mg.
42. **Cheese, camembert :** 300 mg.

43. **8% protein curd:** 300 mg.

44. **Cornmeal, white, self-rising, bolted, with wheat flour added, enriched:** 299 mg.

45. **Raw Galician cabbage:** 290 mg.

46. **Milk, canned, condensed, sweetened:** 284 mg.

47. **Fish, salmon, pink, canned, drained solids:** 283 mg.

48. **Kanpyo, (dried gourd strips):** 280 mg.

49. **Milk, dry, nonfat, calcium reduced:** 280 mg.

50. **Cheese, ricotta, part skim milk:** 272 mg.

51. **Almond, kernel, with skin:** 270 mg.

52. **Nuts, almonds, dry roasted, without salt added:** 268 mg.

53. **Cooked cauliflower:** 260 mg.

54. **Soy, low-fat flour:** 260 mg.

55. **Onions, dehydrated flakes:** 257 mg.

56. **Wheat flour, white, all-purpose, enriched, calcium-fortified:** 252 mg.

57. **Soybeans, dried, raw:** 250 mg.

58. **Hazelnut, kernel:** 250 mg.

59. **Bread, cornbread, prepared from recipe, made with low fat (2%) milk:** 249 mg.

60. **Fish, mackerel, jack, canned, drained solids:** 241 mg.

61. **Dry fig:** 240 mg.

62. **Amaranth leaves, cooked, boiled, drained, without salt:** 209 mg.

63. **Cheese, Ricotta, whole milk:** 207 mg.

64. **Collards, frozen, chopped, unprepared:** 201 mg.

65. **Raw parsley:** 200 mg.

66. **Raw cress:** 200 mg.

67. <u>Soybeans, green, raw:</u> 197

68. **Milk, sheep, fluid:** 190 mg.

69. **Yogurt, plain, low fat, 12 grams protein per 8 ounces:** 183 mg.

70. <u>Garlic, raw:</u> 181 mg.

71. <u>Raw white beans:</u> 180 mg.

72. <u>Beef cube for broth:</u> 180 mg.

73. <u>Soluble coffee (powder) with caffeine:</u> 170 mg.

74. <u>Raw butter beans:</u> 170 mg.

75. <u>Seeds, lotus seeds, dried:</u> 163 mg.

76. <u>Bread, reduced-calorie, wheat:</u> 163 mg.

77. <u>Bread, whole-wheat, commercially prepared:</u> 161 mg.

78. <u>Arugula, raw:</u> 160 mg.

79. <u>Fried eel:</u> 160 mg.

80. <u>Turnip greens, frozen, cooked, boiled, drained, without salt:</u> 152 mg.

81. <u>Kale, raw:</u> 150 mg.

82. **Raw goat's milk:** 150 mg.

83. <u>Raw cabbage greens:</u> 150 mg.

84. <u>Seeds, sesame flour, low-fat:</u> 149 mg.

85. <u>Soybeans, green, cooked, boiled, drained, without salt:</u> 145 mg.

86. **Milk, lean, 2% milk fat, fortified with protein, with added vitamin A and vitamin D:** 143 mg.

87. **Milk, skim, 1% fat, fortified with protein, with added vitamin A and vitamin D:** 142 mg.

88. <u>Chickpeas, raw:</u> 140 mg.

89. <u>Roasted and salted pistachio:</u> 140 mg.

90. **Corn flour, yellow, masa, enriched:** 138 mg.

91. **Turnip greens, cooked, boiled, drained, without salt:** 137 mg.

92. **Kale, frozen:** 136 mg.

93. **Bread, cornbread, dry mix, prepared with 2% milk, 80% margarine, and eggs:** 135 mg.

94. **Peppers, sweet, green, freeze-dried:** 134 mg.

95. **Red bean, raw:** 130 mg.

96. **Eggnog:** 130 mg.

97. **Cowpeas (blackeyes), immature seeds, cooked, boiled, drained, without salt:** 128 mg.

98. **Cowpeas (blackeyes), immature seeds, raw:** 126 mg.

99. **Bread, wheat:** 125 mg.

100. **Beans, black, mature seeds, raw:** 123 mg.

101. **Bread, white, commercially prepared, toasted:** 119 mg.

102. **Milk, producer, fluid, 3.7% milkfat:** 119 mg.

103. **Cheese, neufchatel:** 117 mg.

104. **Beet greens, raw:** 117 mg.

105. **Mollusks, oyster, eastern, wild, cooked, moist heat:** 116 mg.

106. **Bread, reduced-calorie, oatmeal:** 115 mg.

107. **Nuts, hazelnuts or filberts:** 114 mg.

108. **Cheese, cottage, lowfat, 2% milkfat:** 111 mg.

109. **Broccoli raab, raw:** 108 mg.

110. **Cream, fluid, half and half:** 107 mg.

111. **Bread, wheat germ, toasted:** 100 mg.

112. **Spinach, raw:** 99 mg.

Appendix D

Detailed Explanation of Each of 22 Key Blood and Urine Tests and Information on How to Interpret Your Results and Adjust the Protocol Accordingly

When it comes to supplementing with high doses of vitamin D, there are a few parameters that you should pay special attention to. Dr. Coimbra states more than twenty of them to which we added the ionogram. In this Appendix, our goal is to understand more deeply what is involved in each of these blood and urine tests and how to interpret our results. Except when otherwise noted, these tests will not require fasting.

As discussed in Chapter 5, we will explore the following tests:

Important Note: The reference values given here are not universal and may vary depending on the method used by the laboratory where the tests are performed. **You should always use the reference values provided by the laboratory** — usually, these values will be in the right-hand column, in the row corresponding to the result.

Vitamin B12 — also known as cyanocobalamin

Reference values:
- Between 180 and 914 ng/L[181]

Vitamin B12 is essential for the correct functioning of the nervous system. The lack of this essential vitamin causes dementia symptoms that can be confused with other better-known diseases such as Alzheimer's.

Vitamin B12 deficiency can get so serious as to cause psychotic problems and concentration deficits higher than those caused by Alzheimer's. However, vitamin B12 deficiency does not cause the pattern of language problems and apraxia characteristic of Alzheimer's disease.

The apraxia is characterized by an inability to perform gestures. It is as if all the brain machinery responsible for the execution of movements was damaged.

Dementia caused by insufficient vitamin B12 may be reversible with adequate vitamin B12 supplementation.[182] Dementia associated with Alzheimer's disease isn't curable, although high doses of vitamin D appear to have a connection with improved cognition[183] possibly even more when combined with curcumin.[184] Positive results have also been found when supplementing with melatonin.[185]

However, dementia is one of the last symptoms of vitamin B12 deficiency. Being essential for the proper functioning of red blood cells, vitamin B12 deficiency causes a type of anemia called pernicious anemia, which leads to death unless the person receives adequate supplementation, usually through intramuscular injections.

In addition, the deficiency of this vitamin causes paresthesia, a type of pain that involves burn and electric shock sensations and tremors. These symptoms are like those caused by the destruction of the myelin sheets that occurs in multiple sclerosis.

In this regard, it's essential to ensure that vitamin B12 levels are well within the reference levels. This is especially important given the ease with which someone can become deficient. Just like with vitamin D, vitamin B12 absorption and metabolization involves many steps and these can be affected by the drugs you take or the quality of your digestive system and diet.

On diet, it's noteworthy that, in addition to cereals and other fortified foods, vitamin B12 is found mainly in animal products. Contrary to popular belief, however, vitamin B12 isn't unique to these foods, being also found in nori, in some algae and mushrooms, and in tempeh — a type of fermented soy.[186, 187]

In case of a deficiency, in addition to intramuscular injections, the patient may opt for oral supplementation. Here, I strongly recommend methylcobalamin to be chosen instead of cyanocobalamin. The difference between the two is like the difference between vitamin D3 and vitamin D2. Methylcobalamin requires fewer metabolization steps to become usable by our organism.

Vitamin B12 is directly related to folic acid. Both folic acid and vitamin B12 are included in the daily supplements recommended by Dr. Coimbra.

Calcitriol — also called 1.25(OH)2 D3, and 1.25-dihydroxycholecalciferol

Reference Values:[188]

- under 16 years: 24–86 pg/mL.
- greater than or equal to 16 years: 18–64 pg/mL.
- with significant variations depending on the chosen laboratory.[189]

Calcitriol is the active form of vitamin D. It is measured to see if the kidneys are fulfilling their function of converting calcifediol — the inactive form — into the active form.[190] This blood test does not require fasting.

The reference values used as guidelines are based on the common values observed in 95% of the population whose values were previously measured. This means when your results are being evaluated in the laboratory, your values are being compared to the values commonly found in other people. If they are similar, you are considered to be within normal range.[191]

However, being that the majority of the population doesn't lead a healthy lifestyle, the average values used to compute the reference range have been getting worse.

By comparison, studies of calcitriol levels in populations with healthier habits revealed reference values between 19.5 pg/ml and 38.5 pg/ml (29.0 pg/ml ± 9.5 pg/ml).[192] Also, a smaller study of these populations indicated regular values in the order of "23.6 ± 1.3 pg/ml," that is: between 22.3 pg/ml and 24.9 pg/ml.[193, 194]

According to the Mayo Clinic: 'Levels below the reference values are indicative of chronic renal failure and hypoparathyroidism' — an underactive parathyroid gland. 'Elevated levels are indicative of sarcoidosis, granulomatous diseases and some cancers, primary hyperparathyroidism and physiological hyperparathyroidism' — an overactive parathyroid gland.[195]

Sarcoidosis is characterized by the formation of granulomas, small nodules that the immune system creates to isolate invaders, due to the presence of permanent inflammation mainly in the lungs.[196] On the other hand, granulomatous diseases involve disturbances in the immune system.[197]

Sarcoidosis may indicate a hypersensitivity to vitamin D,[198] hence the importance of this blood test.

Calcifediol — also called Calcidiol, 25(OH)D3, 25(OH)D and 25-hydroxycholecalciferol

Calcifediol, or 25 (OH) D3, is the blood test commonly used to determine whether a person is deficient in vitamin D and does not require fasting.

Reference values according to the Brazilian Society of Clinical Pathology and the Brazilian Society of Endocrinology and Metabolism:

- Above 20 ng/mL is the desired value.
- Between 30 and 60 ng/mL is the recommended value for groups at risk like the elderly, pregnant women, infants, patients with rickets/osteomalacia, osteoporosis, patients with a history of falls and fractures, secondary causes of osteoporosis (diseases and medications), hyperparathyroidism, inflammatory diseases, autoimmune diseases, chronic kidney disease and malabsorption syndromes (clinical or post-surgical). "
- Above 100 ng/mL carries the risk of toxicity and hypercalcemia.[199]

These ranges are very similar to those referenced worldwide.

Mayo Clinic, in its official website, provides the following reference ranges:[200]

- Less than 10 ng/mL — severe deficiency.
- Between 10-19 ng/mL — mild to moderate deficiency.
- Between 20-50 ng/mL — optimum levels.
- Between 51-80 ng/mL — increased risk of hypercalciuria.
- Higher than 80 ng/mL — toxicity possible.

The vitamin D council, on the other hand, gives the following recommendations and warnings:

"A 25(OH)D level determines whether a person is deficient, sufficient, or toxic in vitamin D. At this time, there is not a consensus in medicine in what blood levels define these categories.

The Vitamin D Council recommends maintaining serum levels of 50 ng/ml (equivalent to 125 nmol/L), with the following reference ranges:

- Deficient: 0-40 ng/ml (0-100 nmol/l)
- Sufficient: 40-80 ng/ml (100-200 nmol/l)
- High Normal: 80-100 ng/ml (200-250 nmol/l)
- Undesirable: > 100 ng/ml (> 250 nmol/l)
- Toxic: > 150 ng/ml (> 375 nmol/l)"[201]

How can we make sense of this varying reference ranges?

As pointed out by Dr. Coimbra, the factor that interests us is whether the body is actually using this circulating vitamin D.

It's similar to what happens with insulin: you may have an acceptable amount of circulating insulin, but it won't do you much good if your cells have become resistant to it. In these circumstances, it may even need injectable insulin to overcome this resistance.

Similarly, if your body is making a proper use of the circulating vitamin D this will be reflected in your PTH levels — analyzed below. So, the values of calcifediol — vitamin D — serve mostly the purpose of helping you gauge your risk of developing hypercalcemia.

For example, suppose your blood test reveals vitamin D levels above 100 ng/mL. This means that you are at risk of hypercalcemia. However, suppose that even with these levels, your PTH values are not at the desired low level. This indicates that although vitamin D may be stimulating your bones to release calcium into the blood and encouraging your intestine to increase calcium absorption, the truth is **the amount of vitamin D is not yet high enough to overcome the resistance of your organism**.

Another possibility for high levels of circulating vitamin D and an unresponsive PTH level involves difficulties in the metabolism of vitamin B2.

In any case, you would have to continue increasing your vitamin D intake to increasingly potential dangerous levels — due to the higher risk of hypercalcemia. Then you would have to take even more care to comply with the safety measures: (1) to avoid milk and milk by-products because of their high calcium content, (2) to drink at least 2.5 liters of fluids a day, (3) to use an Herbensurina like tea, (4) to exercise — thus stimulates your bones to reabsorb calcium — and (5) to take your vitamin K2 in appropriate amounts. In addition with (6) more regular blood calcium and renal function tests.

In these cases of high resistance to the immunomodulatory effects of vitamin D specialized medical follow-up would be essential. Why is the case? Because these people would need to reach circulating levels of vitamin D in the range of the thousands of ng/mL until their PTH finally drops to the desired low level.

PTH — also known as Parathyroid Hormone or Parathormone

Reference values:
- Between 10 and 65 pg/mL or 10 and 65 ng/L[202]

Here lies the *pièce de résistance* (cornerstone) of the whole therapy: lowering PTH, without, however, allowing it to drop below the lower end of the reference range. For a laboratory using a reference range between 10.0 and 65.0 pg/mL, this would mean preventing PTH from dropping below 10.0 pg/mL while attempting to get it as close as possible to that value.

PTH is secreted with the goal of raising blood calcium levels. If calcium is high, PTH is expected to be low. A physician, usually an endocrinologist, uses his knowledge of this relationship between PTH and calcium to define the health status of your parathyroid gland.

On the one hand, *high* blood calcium should be interpreted by the parathyroid gland as a signal to produce *less* PTH. Thus, if calcium and PTH are both elevated this may be indicative of hyperparathyroidism — an overactive parathyroid gland.

On the other hand, if blood calcium levels are *low* and PTH is *not high* this is also a bad sign. Low levels of both calcium and PTH may indicate hypoparathyroidism — an underactive parathyroid gland.

This allows us to understand why specialized medical monitoring is vital, especially in the cases where dosages above 40,000 IU of daily vitamin D are used.

This is because a measurement of circulating PTH is only useful to the extent that the other factors influencing PTH are under control. For example, a diet that is extremely deficient in calcium would cause a decrease in calcium blood levels, even in the presence of high doses of vitamin D. This would cause PTH to increase *for that reason*.

On the other hand, a calcium–rich diet would increase calcium levels, especially due to the presence of high doses of vitamin D. This would cause a significant reduction in PTH production. You would think your PTH was lowering due to vitamin D when in fact it was dropping as a reaction to the raising calcium levels.

This allows us to see just how important the dietary restrictions are. **Only if there's a low calcium intake and there is no evidence of parathyroid disease, can any changes in PTH levels be attributed to vitamin D.**

Calcium (total and ionized)

Reference ranges as reported by medscape.com:[203]

Total Calcium in Men:
- Younger than 12 months: Not established
- Age 1–14 years: 9.6–10.6 mg/dL
- Age 15–16 years: 9.5–10.5 mg/dL
- Age 17–18 years: 9.5–10.4 mg/dL
- Age 19–21 years: 9.3–10.3 mg/dL
- Age 22 years and older: 8.9–10.1 mg/dL

Total calcium in women:
- Younger than 12 months: Not established
- Age 1–11 years: 9.6–10.6 mg/dL
- Age 12–14 years: 9.5–10.4 mg/dL
- Age 15–18 years: 9.1–10.3 mg/dL
- Age 19 years and older: 8.9–10.1 mg/dL

Ionized calcium in men:
- Younger than 12 months: Not established
- 1–19 years: 5.1–5.9 mg/dL
- Age 20 years and older: 4.8–5.7 mg/dL

Ionized calcium in women:
- Younger than 12 months: Not established
- 1–17 years: 5.1–5.9 mg/dL
- Age 18 years and older: 4.8–5.7 mg/dL

99% of our calcium is stored in our bones, while the remaining 1% is in the blood, soft tissues and extracellular space.[204]

However, not all the calcium circulating in our blood is free — or ionized. Nearly half of our blood calcium is connected to albumin and other compounds and is inactive.[205] Hence the importance of measuring total calcium as well.

These blood tests are critical in evaluating any potential vitamin D toxicity before the onset of hypercalcemia.

When these tests reveal levels **above** the reference range, a healthcare professional must be consulted because you are in a high risk of developing hypercalcemia. Higher than expected calcium levels may also indicate renal issues or endocrine problems. In any case, calcium levels above the reference range will tell you that your organism may not be responding well to the protocol and the root cause needs to be investigated and treated since it may involve your bones, kidneys, parathyroid gland or another organ.

Urea (BUN — *Blood Urea Nitrogen)*

Reference range for blood urea nitrogen:

- Between 6 and 20 mg of urea nitrogen per 100 mL[206] — equivalent to 13 mg and 43 mg of urea, respectively.[207]

BUN aims to directly assess renal function. It measures the blood values of some of the molecules filtered by our kidneys. High values are a red alert of reduced renal function.

Certain drugs may interfere with your BUN results. This means that it is necessary to receive medical advice on how to prepare for the test, especially if you are taking drugs that can't be stopped without medical supervision, even if for only a few days.

In addition, a diet either rich or deficient in protein will affect your results. For this reason, BUN and creatinine are frequently done together. Creatinine is discussed below.

Creatinine

Reference values:[208]

- Adult males: Between 0.5 and 1.2 mg/dL
- Adult females: Between 0.4 and 1.1 mg/dL
- Children (up to 12 years of age): Between 0.0 and 0.7 mg/dL

Creatinine is a molecule present in our muscles. Our kidneys filter more than 7 liters of blood per hour. Creatinine is one of the molecules being constantly filtered. For that reason, if creatinine starts accumulating in our blood and we are not a young and muscular athlete this is a warning sign. Values well above 1.2 mg/dl are a strong indication of kidney disease.

Since the BUN is a test whose results may be influenced by a diet that is either low or rich in protein, drugs or other factors, creatinine ends up being an ally in the validation of the BUN result.

Creatinine concentration reflects how effective our kidney is in filtering our blood.

In the case of someone taking high doses of vitamin D, higher creatinine levels are a red alert that can't be ignored. If the kidney is not working properly, the person is risking further damage and hypercalcemia. Tighter medical supervision becomes mandatory.

Albumin

Reference values:

- 3.5 to 5.5 g/dL (i.e. 35–55 g/L). A value that can vary from laboratory to laboratory.[209, 210]

Albumin is the most abundant protein in the human blood. High values indicate a state of dehydration. Low values, on the other hand, can indicate problems in the liver because this protein is synthesized there.

In our blood, albumin acts as a carrier, transporting hormones and other molecules. Each hormone has a specific carrier. However, when these become saturated, albumin comes to the rescue, compensating for the lack of available specialized carriers.

Another important function of albumin is in providing us with raw building materials. Being a very versatile protein, albumin is used by the body as an internal source of amino acids. Amino acids are the building blocks used for, for example, building muscle and skin. Because of this, albumin is vital in healing burns and wounds.

Therefore, after suffering such a trauma, it's natural to see a decrease in serum albumin levels. The same would happen in a low protein diet because you wouldn't be giving your body the proteins it required to build albumin.

Albumin levels also give us a glimpse of how the liver is doing. Testing BUN, creatinine, and albumin levels give the doctor an even more accurate perspective on the health status of the kidneys. Especially if, in addition to a blood test, a urine albumin test is also performed. Why? Because elevated amounts of albumin in the urine would indicate that the kidney filtration system isn't working properly.

Ferritin

Reference values:[211]

- Men: Between 23.0 and 336.0 ng/mL.
- Women: Between 11.0 and 306.0 ng/mL.

Iron is an essential mineral. It's used in the construction of hemoglobin. Hemoglobin is a protein that exists in our red blood cells, being responsible for proving red blood cells with the ability to transport oxygen. This means that without iron our blood would be unable to transport sufficient amounts of oxygen.

As such, our body must ensure that iron is available at all times. But there is a problem. Excess iron is toxic, so our body can't simply allow the extra iron to circulate freely through the blood. How can we solve this problem? With ferritin. Ferritin is a ball-shaped molecule that surrounds iron atoms. Within each ferritin protein sphere, we can find up to 4,500 iron atoms,[212] isolated and unable to intoxicate us.

Ferritin, in turn, is kept stored, especially in the liver, ready to release its iron reserves as soon as they are needed.

Ferritin tests help us not only in keeping track of ferritin reserves but also in measuring inflammation. This is because inflammatory diseases cause an increase in ferritin levels. Along with the remaining tests, ferritin is useful in giving us an overall picture of an individual's health and nutritional status.

This test doesn't require fasting and an extended fast may even affect the results.

Chromium (serum)

Reference values:

- Less than 0.3 ng/L when proper testing procedures are followed by the blood analyst.[213]

Like iron, chromium is another mineral that becomes toxic when present in excessive amounts. However, there are two important differences.

First, unlike iron, our body does not have a safe storage system for chromium.

In addition, although chromium has been unanimously considered an essential mineral for decades,[214] in recent times its status of "essential mineral" has been called into question.[215] Despite this, this mineral has been shown to be pharmacologically active in certain animal clinical studies.[216] Even so, its ability to exert an effect on the human body has not yet gained unequivocal approval from the scientific community.[217]

Still, there are clinical studies demonstrating its positive effect on the human glucose metabolism.[218, 219] For example, in *Clinical studies on chromium picolinate supplementation in diabetes mellitus — a review*, the conclusion of the researchers, after reviewing 15 studies, was as follows:

"All 15 studies showed salutary effects in at least one parameter of diabetes management, including dyslipidemia. Positive outcomes from [chromium picolinate] supplementation included reduced blood glucose, insulin, cholesterol, and triglyceride levels and reduced requirements for hypoglycemic medication." And: "The pooled data from studies using [chromium picolinate] supplementation for type 2 diabetes mellitus subjects show substantial reductions in hyperglycemia and hyperinsulinemia, which equate to a reduced risk for disease complications. Collectively, the data support the safety and therapeutic value of [chromium picolinate] for the management of cholesterolemia and hyperglycemia in subjects with diabetes."[220]

It is clear why chromium picolinate is recommended by Dr. Coimbra in its protocol, even amongst the controversy within the scientific community as to whether chromium is an essential mineral.

However, because of the toxic potential of this substance when in excess, it makes sense to keep tight control over its blood levels.

This is especially important given how chromium toxicity manifests itself in renal function.[221]

As noted, the kidneys are our greatest ally against excess calcium in the blood. We want our kidneys to maintain their filtering and excretory capacities at the highest possible level. Therefore, if you are taking chromium picolinate it is essential to keep up to date on the levels of this mineral in your blood.

Phosphate (serum)

Reference values:[222]

Men:
- 1–4 years: Between 4.3 and 5.4 mg/dL
- 5–13 years: Between 3.7 and 5.4 mg/dL
- 14–15 years: Between 3.5 and 5.3 mg/dL
- 16–17 years: Between 3.1 and 4.7 mg/dL
- 18 years and older: Between 2.5 and 4.5 mg/dL

Women:
- 1–7 years: Between 4.3 and 5.4 mg/dL
- 8–13 years: Between 4.0 and 5.2 mg/dL
- 14–15 years: Between 3.5 and 4.9 mg/dL
- 16–17 years: Between 3.1 and 4.7 mg/dL
- 18 years and older: Between 2.5 and 4.5 mg/dL

Phosphate results from the reaction between phosphorus and oxygen. In humans, this molecule is found in abundance in the bones. Because of this, the regulation of phosphate levels depends on the interaction between our bones and our excretory channels: the kidneys and the intestine.

As such, elevated phosphate levels in our blood indicate kidney problems.

In addition, phosphate levels are directly related to vitamin D levels and parathyroid gland function. High values may indicate hypoparathyroidism and low values may indicate the opposite problem, hyperparathyroidism.

When both calcium and phosphate levels rise they can lead to calcium phosphate deposits in various parts of the body.

Elevated levels of vitamin D increase the absorption of both calcium and phosphorus, potentially overworking the kidneys. Therefore, this blood test is intended to ensure an accurate monitoring of kidney function during high-dose vitamin D therapy.

Ammonia (serum)

Reference values:
- Between 15 and 45 µ/dL
- Equivalent to: Between 11 and 32 µmol/L223

Ammonia is toxic to our brain. However, before reaching the brain it needs to cross the blood–brain barrier. This barrier acts as a military checkpoint and ammonia is not on their list. This is very reassuring. Why? Because ammonia causes mental confusion, drowsiness, and may even induce coma and death!

However, our body is in constant contact with ammonia. Ammonia is one of the byproducts of protein digestion. In addition, ammonia is also produced by our gut bacteria.

For these reasons our body is well equipped to deal with ammonia, preventing it from accumulating in the blood. How? First, the liver processes the ammonia, transforming it into urea. Then the kidneys expel this urea.

But if there is any disturbance in this cycle ammonia begins to accumulate in our blood. The more it accumulates the greater the likelihood that some ammonia will eventually cross the blood–brain barrier.

Because of this, and especially in a therapy with high doses of vitamin D, awareness of blood ammonia levels is one more way to ensure close monitoring of renal and hepatic function.

Complete amino acid profile

Reference values, when 18 years or older, according to the Mayo Clinic:[224]

- **Urine, in nmol/mg creatinine:**

  - 1–Methylhistidine: between 23 and 1339
  - 3–Methylhistidine: between 70 and 246
  - *Alanine: between 56 and 518*
  - Allo–isoleucine: less than 7
  - Alpha–amino–n–butyric Acid: less than 19
  - Alpha–aminoadipic Acid: less than 47
  - Anserine: less than 38
  - *Arginine: less than 114*
  - Argininosuccinic Acid: less than 15
  - Asparagine: between 25 and 238
  - *Aspartic Acid: less than 10*
  - Beta–Alanine: less than 52
  - Beta–aminoisobutyric Acid: less than 301
  - Carnosine: less than 35
  - Citrulline: less than 12
  - Cystathionine: less than 30
  - *Cystine: between 10 and 98*
  - Ethanolamine: between 95 and 471
  - Gamma Amino–n–butyric Acid: less than 5
  - *Glutamic Acid: less than 34*
  - *Glutamine: between 93 and 686*
  - *Glycine: between 229 and 2989*
  - *Histidine: between 81 and 1128*
  - Homocitrulline: less than 30
  - Hydroxylysine: less than 12
  - Hydroxyproline: less than 15
  - **Isoleucine: less than 22**
  - **Leucine: less than 51**
  - **Lysine: between 15 and 271**
  - **Methionine: less than 16**

- Ornithine: less than 25
- **Phenylalanine: between 13 and 70**
- Phosphoethanolamine: less than 48
- Phosphoserine: less than 1
- *Proline: less than 26*
- Sarcosine: less than 3
- *Serine: between 97 and 540*
- Taurine: between 24 and 1531
- **Threonine: between 31 and 278**
- **Tryptophan: between 18 and 114**
- *Tyrosine: between 15 and 115*
- **Valine: between 11 and 61**

- **Plasma, in nmol/mg:**[225]

  - 1-Methylhistidine: less than 28.
  - 3-Methylhistidine: between 2 and 9.
  - *Alanine: between 200 and 579.*
  - Allo-isoleucine: less than 5.
  - Alpha-amino-n-butyric Acid: between 9 and 37.
  - Alpha-aminoadipic Acid: less than 3.
  - Anserine: less than 1.
  - *Arginine: between 32 and 120.*
  - Argininosuccinic Acid: less than 2.
  - Asparagine: between 37 and 92.
  - *Aspartic Acid: less than 7.*
  - Beta-Alanine: less than 29.
  - Beta-aminoisobutyric Acid: less than 5.
  - Carnosine: less than 1.
  - Citrulline: between 17 and 46.
  - Cystathionine: less than 5.
  - *Cystine: between 3 and 95.*
  - Ethanolamine: less than 67.
  - Gamma Amino-n-butyric Acid: less than 2.
  - *Glutamic Acid: between 13 and 113.*
  - *Glutamine: between 371 and 957.*
  - *Glycine: between 126 and 490.*

- *Histidine: between 39 and 123.*
- Homocitrulline: less than 2.
- Hydroxylysine: less than 2.
- Hydroxyproline: between 4 and 29.
- **Isoleucine: between 36 and 107.**
- **Leucine: between 68 and 183.**
- **Lysine: between 103 and 255.**
- **Methionine: between 4 and 44.**
- Ornithine: between 38 and 130.
- **Phenylalanine: between 35 and 80.**
- Phosphoethanolamine: less than 12.
- Phosphoserine: less than 18.
- *Proline: between 97 and 368.*
- Sarcosine: less than 5.
- *Serine: between 63 and 187.*
- Taurine: between 42 and 156.
- **Threonine: between 85 and 231.**
- **Tryptophan: between 29 and 77.**
- *Tyrosine: between 31 and 90.*
- **Valine: between 136 and 309.**

Amino acids are the basic constituents of proteins. We can imagine children playing with blocks. Depending on how these blocks are stacked, we may end up building a house, a bus or a train. Amino acids are like these blocks.

Each amino acid has a different shape and depending on how they are assembled together, they can be used to produce countless different types of proteins.

Our body can manufacture some of these blocks. These are called nonessential amino acids. They are aspartic acid, glutamic acid, alanine, arginine, asparagine, cysteine, glycine, glutamine, histidine, proline, serine and tyrosine — in italics.

There are other amino acids our body is unable to manufacture these are known as essential amino acids. These are valine, threonine, tryptophan, methionine, phenylalanine, lysine, isoleucine and leucine — in bold.

The remaining amino acids can be classified as non–essential and are not given the same attention from a nutrition perspective. They have, nevertheless, scientific interest. For example, sarcosine is formed by our body in the metabolism of other amino acids and is measured with the goal of evaluating the progress of prostate cancer.[226]

Amino acids can be measured in plasma or urine. Plasma amino acid concentrations vary by about 30% throughout the day, being higher in the middle of the afternoon and lower in the morning.[227] This is one of the reasons why urine measurement is preferred. However, certain circumstances, such as the presence of blood in the urine, make urine measurements unreliable.

From laboratory to laboratory reference ranges vary, as well as the specific number of amino acids tested. This is a fairly expensive exam due to the number of parameters examined. However, if you choose to get your amino acid profile examined you will get an excellent sense of the state of your body with respect to the absorption and metabolism of the various amino acids.

Talk to your doctor before choosing to perform this exam so that he can instruct you on what parameters are needed in your case — if any.

ALT — also called alanine aminotransferase, alanine transaminase and glutamic pyruvic transaminase or TGP

Reference values:
- From 7 to 55 units per liter (U/L)[228]

ALT is an enzyme — a molecule that helps the body perform chemical reactions. It's present primarily in our liver and kidneys,[229] and also in our heart and muscles.

When any of these organs are damaged, cells rupture and ALT is released into the blood. Thus, high ALT values indicate some of these organs have been damaged, with one of the prime suspects being the liver. But how can we know for sure?

To assist in doing this "chemical triangulation," ALT is often examined along with another molecule: AST. In the next page, we will look at AST.

AST — aspartate aminotransferase, also called glutamic oxaloacetic transaminase or ORT

Reference range:
- From 8 to 48 units per liter (U/L)[230]

Like ALT, AST is a vital enzyme present in the liver and in other organs. When both ALT and AST are high this is a strong warning that the liver may be sick. At this point, your doctor will prescribe additional tests to confirm his suspicions.

In turn, low values may be indicative of a deficiency in vitamin B6. This is especially noticeable in hospitalized patients who, due to their fragility, tend to develop a vitamin B6 deficiency.[231]

TSH — Thyroid stimulating hormone

Reference values:[232]

- Children:
    - Birth to 4 days: Between 1 and 39 mIU/L
    - 2 to 20 weeks: Between 1.7 and 9.1 mIU/L
    - 21 weeks to 20 years: Between 0.7 and 64 mIU/L

- Adults:
    - Between 21 and 54 years: Between 0.4 and 4.2 mIU/L
    - Between 55 and 87 years: Between 0.5 and 8.9 mIU/L

- Women, during Pregnancy:
    - First trimester: Between 0.3-4.5 mIU/L
    - Second trimester: Between 0.5 and 4.6 mIU/L
    - Third trimester: Between 0.8 and 5.2 mIU/L

Thyroid stimulating hormone (TSH), as the name implies, is a hormone that stimulates our thyroid to work. Our thyroid is responsible for sending messages — hormones — that regulate our whole body. These hormones, T3 and T4, regulate the way we turn nutrients into energy.

Two common problems affecting the thyroid are hyperthyroidism and hypothyroidism. As the prefixes "hyper" and "hypo" indicate, in hyperthyroidism the thyroid works too much and in hypothyroidism, less than it should.

To tame this gland, our body uses TSH.

TSH is produced by the pituitary gland, which is located in the lower part of our brain. When the thyroid is overworking, TSH levels in the blood go down. In turn, if the thyroid is working less than it should, the TSH levels are increased.

We can compare this with what happens when we are driving our car. If the car is going too slow, we'll press on the gas pedal.

But, if the car accelerates too much, we'll take our foot off the accelerator.

TSH is the gas pedal. When the thyroid starts having problems and working less than it was supposed to, our body presses on the accelerator and keeps sending TSH — messengers after messengers demanding the thyroid to work more. These elevated levels are not normal, and this alerts the doctor to the likely underlying issue: hypothyroidism.

On the other hand, if the thyroid is working too hard, our body takes its foot off the gas pedal, lowering TSH. Thus, low levels of TSH are indicative of an overactive thyroid.

For this blood test, a fasting of 3 hours is recommended.[233]

This exam is important because **an overactive thyroid will cause hypercalcemia in about 1 in 5 people.**[234] This means hyperthyroidism can give you a false impression that your PTH has gone down because you are reaching an optimal level of vitamin D supplementation, when in fact it was just the parathyroid reacting to the elevated calcium levels by lowering PTH production.

The inverse relationship, that an underactive thyroid gland in a state of hypothyroidism, influences the parathyroid gland to produce more PTH is not well established in humans with functional kidneys.[235, 236]

Serum alkaline phosphatase (specific bone fraction)

Reference values:[237]

- Men:
  - Less than 2 years: 25–221 mcg/L
  - Between 2 and 9 years: 27–148 mcg/L
  - Between 10–13 years: 35–169 mcg/L
  - Between 14–17 years: 13–111 mcg/L
  - 18 years or older: Less than or equal to 20 mcg/L

- Women:
  - Less than 2 years: 28–187 mcg/L
  - Between 2–9 years: 31–152 mcg/L
  - Between 10–13 years: 29–177 mcg/L
  - Between 14–17 years: 7–41 mcg/L
  - 18 years or older and premenopausal: Less than or equal to 14 mcg/L
  - 18 years or older and postmenopausal: Less than or equal to 22 mcg/L

Our bones are living networks in constant remodeling. One of the cells responsible for the formation of bone tissue is called osteoblast. To fulfill its function, the osteoblast constructs diverse substances, one of them is called alkaline phosphatase.

Alkaline phosphatase is an enzyme that is present throughout the body and has several functions. When it's produced by the osteoblast it helps the minerals to bond to the bone. We can imagine the osteoblast as a bricklayer doing mortar — alkaline phosphatase — and using this mortar to join calcium and other minerals to form bone tissue.[238]

Now, imagine getting to a construction site and finding out that very little mortar is being made. What would be your conclusion? The mortar is essential for bonding bricks and making solid walls. So, if there is a problem with the mortar, the whole structure is at risk.

Similarly, if a blood test of the bone fraction of alkaline phosphatase reveals very low values this may indicate a skeletal problem such as osteoporosis.

Also, if you notice the variations in the reference range, you will realize that while a person is growing up there are higher levels of this substance in the blood. This is because this is the period when the skeleton is increasing in volume daily. On the other hand, as the person enters adulthood, the production of bone decreases because the skeleton will no longer significantly increase in volume.

Low values of alkaline phosphatase are also indicative of vitamin D deficiency.

High levels, in turn, indicate abnormal bone activity. Unfortunately, this may be a sign of bone cancer, requiring more specific tests before reaching a definitive diagnosis.

Serum P1NP (intact N-terminal propeptide of type 1 collagen), collected 2 hours after getting up

Reference values:[239]

- Men over 18 years of age: 22–87 mcg/L
- Pre-menopausal women 18 years and over: Between 19 and 83 mcg/L
- Postmenopausal women 18 years and older: Between 16 and 96 mcg/L

To understand the relevance of an analysis to P1NP we first must understand what collagen is.

Collagen is a protein used in the construction of various structures like skin, tendons and bones. For this reason, some collagen–based creams are used to help the skin recover from wounds.[240] Collagen is also used as a beauty cream.

There are at least 18 types of collagen.[241] The most abundant in bone is type 1 collagen. This type of collagen is one of the chemicals produced by the osteoblast during the formation of bone tissue.

It just so happens that during the formation of collagen the osteoblast attaches some molecules, called propeptides, at the ends of the collagen. When this happens, a new substance, procollagen, is formed.

A propeptide is an inactive molecule. However, that does not mean it's useless. It just means that if you want to make it useful you need to either break it apart or attach it to another molecule.

We can compare what happens to collagen with what happens to a television set in a TV factory. After producing the television set, the workers insert foam plates on top and underneath it. These foam plates are shaped like a TV set and fit in perfectly. However, by themselves, these plates are not useful.

Now imagine that you want to know how many televisions the factory is producing. You may decide to count either the televisions or the foam plates.

It's the same with collagen. If you want to get a sense of how well osteoblasts are working you can do so by measuring the propeptides they are attaching to collagen.

One of these is the propeptide of type 1 collagen, that is, one of the molecules that is embedded at the end of type 1 collagen — also changing its name from "collagen" to "procollagen." And as it turns out, some of these propeptides end up in the bloodstream where they can then be measured.

Elevated P1NP values indicate that the osteoblasts are very busy making bone. Again, this can be a bad sign. For example, in patients with breast cancer, elevated P1NP values are a poor prognosis as to whether bone metastases are present or not.[242]

However, elevated P1NP values are normal when the body is recovering from a bone fracture or during normal skeletal development.

In addition, since P1NP is excreted by the kidneys, high values may also be indicative of renal problems.

Finally, in addition to its role in monitoring osteoporosis, P1NP is also an extra diagnostic tool for assessing parathyroid gland problems.

Serum CTX (C-terminal telopeptide)

Reference values:[243]

- Men:
    - 30 to 50 years: Between 0.016 and 0.584 ng / ml.
    - from 50 to 70 years: Less than 0.704 ng / ml.
    - over 70 years: Less than 0,854 ng / ml.

- Women:
    - Pre-menopausal: Between 0.025 and 0.573 ng / ml.
    - Postmenopausal: Between 0.104 and 1.008 ng / ml.

In addition to the osteoblast, which specializes in bone formation, the body also has cells specialized in bone tissue removal. These cells are called osteoclasts.

If we imagine osteoblasts as masons and builders, we can imagine osteoclasts as the demolition team. (Check the footnote for a cool mnemonic)[244]

While the joint measurement of alkaline phosphatase and P1NP gave us a good idea of how the osteoclasts are working to form bone tissue, measuring the C-terminal telopeptide helps us to understand how osteoclasts are performing their function.

In addition, this blood test is very useful when the patient is being treated with bisphosphonates. In addition to their important role in treating bone metastases, bisphosphonates are used to treat hypercalcemia — reducing the level of calcium in the blood.

However, one of the side effects of bisphosphonates is how they affect your jawbone, leading to necrosis — or "rotting" — of this bone structure. This happens because a bisphosphonate will reduce the body's ability to renew bone tissue.

Due to the daily activity of mastication and because of the teeth, the jaw requires constant bone remodeling. Because of this, it makes sense that its bone tissue would be one of the most affected by a drug that inhibits bone remodeling.[245, 246]

Thus, elevated C-terminal telopeptide values in patients with osteoporosis are indicative that the disease will progress more rapidly.[247] Along with the remaining exams, this blood test provides a competent doctor with a window into the patient's bone tissues.

Calcium in the urine of 24 hours (with total volume)

Reference values for people with an average calcium intake of 600 to 800 milligrams per day:[248]

- Men: Between 25-300 mg of calcium in the urine of 24 hours.
- Women: Between 20-275 mg of calcium in the urine of 24 hours.
- Hypercalciuria: Over 350 mg of calcium per urine sample.

While very useful, this exam is a bit inconvenient as it requires you to collect your own urine in a jug, or bottle, for an entire day. This container will be provided by the laboratory when you schedule the exam and may take up to 2 liters of urine. Some people may need up to two such containers.

Upon waking up, you should empty your bladder. This first-morning urine will not be stored into the jug. Afterward, all the remaining liquid expelled by your kidneys produce in the next 24 hours should be collected.

As you may imagine, this whole process can become inconvenient. However, you must realize how important this test is. Along with calcifediol (vitamin D), PTH, and blood calcium, this test is one of the four that you should *always* perform.

Why is it so important?

We recall that the goal of high-dose vitamin D therapy is to lower your PTH to the minimum value allowed by the reference range. However, due to the resistance that many organisms have to vitamin D, to achieve this goal, it may be necessary to supplement with a very high daily dose.

There are reported cases of people having to increase their vitamin D dosage to a point where their calcifediol levels were between 300 and 4,000 ng/mL — four thousand nanograms per milliliter![249] Now, if we remember, reaching just 100 ng/mL is enough to produce toxic results in some people.

This toxicity manifests itself as hypercalcemia and your first line of defense against this outcome are your kidneys with their ability to remove excess calcium.

In perspective, collecting 24 hours of urine in a bottle is a tiny unimportant matter.

How should you interpret your results?

If your urine calcium levels are high you need to (1) take even more care not to ingest dairy products, foods fortified with calcium or even bread, (2) ensure that your fluid intake is near the 2.5 daily liters goal (2.64 quarts) and (3) have your daily dose of exercise and vitamin K2. Also include "Herbensurina" type teas — whose contents are again, for your convenience, available in the footnote.[250]

In severe cases of hypercalcemia, bisphosphonates — a drug that only a doctor can prescribe — or other procedures may be used.

On the other hand, low values will also be troublesome. After all, you're hoping your kidneys to be working hard to excrete any excess calcium. This means a low level of calcium in your urine would indicate problems with your kidney function.

Phosphate in the urine of 24 hours (with total volume)

Reference values:

- Less than 1.1 grams in the urine of 24 hours.[251]

As one of the most abundant minerals in our bones, phosphate is one of the minerals that, like calcium, is expected to be released into the blood as both PTH and vitamin D stimulate bone demineralization.

As such, there is a possibility that the phosphorus levels in your blood will increase, causing hyperphosphatemia. This condition, however, is very rare, occurring only in the case of a severe deficiency in renal function.

Blood phosphate testing along with this urine test will give you an even clearer picture of your kidney function during the protocol — or a timely warning that your kidneys need specialized medical attention.

Low levels of phosphate in the urine may indicative of a vitamin D deficiency.

Also, and since bone phosphate is released into the blood in response to PTH, a reduction in phosphate levels in your urine is another indication of a potential hypoparathyroidism.

Ionogram (sodium, potassium, chloride, magnesium and bicarbonate) — also called electrolyte balance and electrolyte profile — and magnesium

Reference values:
Sodium:
- 12 months or older: 135.0 to 145.0 mmol/L.[252]

Potassium:
- 12 months or older: 3.6 to 5.2 mmol/L[253]

Chloride:
- Between 1 and 17 years: 102 to 112 mmol/L
- 18 years and older: 98 to 107 mmol/L.[254]

Magnesium:
- Between 0 and 2 years: 1.6 to 2.7 mg/dL
- Between 3 and 5 years: 1.6 to 2.6 mg/dL
- Between 6 and 8 years: 1.6 to 2.5 mg/dL
- Between 9 and 11 years: 1.6 to 2.4 mg/dL
- Between 12 and 17 years: 1.6 to 2.3 mg/dL
- 17 years and older: 1.7 to 2.3 mg/dL[255]

Bicarbonate:
- Men:
  - Between 12 and 24 months: 17 to 25 mmol/L
  - Between 3 years: 18 to 26 mmol/L
  - Between 4 and 5 years: 19 to 27 mmol/L
  - Between 6 and 7 years: 20 to 28 mmol/L
  - Between 8 and 17 years: 21 to 29 mmol/L
  - 18 years and older: 22 to 29 mmol/L
- Women:
  - Between 1 and 3 years: 18 to 25 mmol/L
  - Between 4 and 5 years: 19 to 26 mmol/L

    o   Between 6 and 7 years: 20 to 27 mmol/L
    o   Between 8 and 9 years: 21 to 28 mmol/L
    o   10 years and older: 22 to 29 mmol/L[256]

The purpose of the ionogram is to measure the blood levels of your electrolytes. Electrolytes are minerals with a positive charge. Or, in other words, they are one of the reasons our body can use electric current at the cellular level, among other vital functions.

For example, sodium, potassium and chloride are responsible for regulating the amount of water inside our cells and bicarbonate regulates the level of acidity in our blood.

Besides these four, there are also two other fairly common electrolytes in our body: phosphorus, considered under "phosphate" and calcium.

If the balance between our electrolytes is disturbed, our body takes steps to correct it quickly. Why?

Sometimes the cell is compared to a city by virtue of all the complex tasks that it performs inside its membrane. Imagine the chaos that would be for a city, like New York, if power grid failures become the norm. Something similar would happen in our organism with electrolyte imbalances.

The consumption of water in large quantities and the extra work being performed by your kidneys creates the possibility of an electrolyte imbalance.

For this reason, the ionogram is a simple, relatively inexpensive and effective way of ensuring any imbalance is readily diagnosed and corrected. This avoids the suffering caused by a serious imbalance, which may include symptoms as severe as dementia, coma, organ failure and death.

Appendix E

Key Insights and Detailed Information on Dosage for Each Recommended Supplement

I n this Appendix we will take a closer look at the benefits, dosages, clinical studies and other indications for the following supplements:

Important note: In the official Coimbra Protocol the dosages and the number of supplements may differ from those presented here because everything is prescribed according to the needs of each patient. These needs are influenced by the type of pathologies the person has, his medical history and the results of his blood tests. You may end up taking supplements that are not listed or not taking supplements that are mentioned here.

As in the rest of the book, every effort was made to ensure that each statement about each supplement was properly referenced by a relevant and current clinical study. This means that it will be easier to recognize the function of each supplement and adapt it to your circumstances.

DHA — Docosahexaenoic Acid

Dose recommended in the protocol: 500 milligrams, 4 times per day.
Best Taken: Along with meals.
Daily total: 2,000 milligrams.

DHA is an essential fatty acid of the omega 3 kind. It turns out that inside our body we have many structures that use fat. As an example, fat is very useful for building up the membranes of our cells.

When we put an oil into water we notice they don't mix. For this reason, we say that fat is hydrophobic. "Hydro" is a word referencing water and "phobic" is related to "phobia." So, when we say that fat is hydrophobic we mean that fat is "afraid" of water.

Now, if you want to put a city in the middle of the water what do you need? You need to build a dam around the city to keep the water out. It turns out that our cells are like cities dipped in extracellular fluid. For the contents of the cell to remain separated from this liquid you need a dam — called a membrane — made of a hydrophobic material — fat.

Without fat, we wouldn't have cells. Fat is *that* important. In fact, our neurons have a lot of it, 60% of our brain is fat.[257]

But not all fat is created equal.

There are some types of fat that our body can't manufacture. These are called essential. We must get them in our diet. One of these essential fats is DHA.

Without enough DHA our brains and our cells don't work as well as they could, especially if you have multiple sclerosis.[258]

But often, we don't consume the amount of DHA we require. How does the body handle this? Being the smart machine that it is, our body turns into a MacGyver of sorts[259] and tries to use other types of fats to repair its membranes. In this way, we can keep ourselves alive but at a loss.

DHA isn't the only essential fat we need, but it's one of the most relevant to our brain. This is noteworthy because, in autoimmune diseases, the brain and the nervous system are often one of the main victims of the unregulated attack of our little white soldiers.

In addition, DHA has anti-inflammatory properties. This means that DHA helps our body reduce the degree of inflammation in the same way an anti-inflammatory drug does. The difference is that DHA doesn't hurt our kidneys. However, with DHA it takes comparatively much more time for the good effects to be felt.

For all this, DHA is one of the supplements recommended by Dr. Coimbra in his protocol.

Another way to supplement DHA along with the other essential fatty acids, such as EPA, is by taking fish oil supplements, such as *krill oil* supplements.

Zinc

Recommended dose in the protocol: 5 milligrams of zinc, 4 times per day.

Best taken: Ideally 1 hour before meals or two hours afterward. But if taking it with an empty stomach causes discomfort you can take it along with food.[260]

Daily total: 20 milligrams.

It is estimated that as many as 2 billion(!) people in the world suffer from retarded growth due to a zinc deficiency. However, and even though it is also essential for the proper functioning of the immune system, it was only in the 1960s that zinc was finally recognized as essential for human life.[261]

Why is it so easy to get deficient in zinc? Because our body doesn't have a system to store it.

Zinc is involved in most immune processes.[262, 263] Thus, zinc supplementation is appropriate and beneficial on its own[264] and as a complement to high-dose vitamin D therapy.

There are several types of zinc available for supplementation purposes, with zinc picolinate being a form that seems to be superior.[265]

Choline

Recommended dose in the protocol: 120 milligrams of choline, 4 times per day.

Best taken according to supplement instructions, with or without food.

Daily total: 480 milligrams.

It was only in 1998 that choline received due recognition as being essential for human health.[266]

It is essential for our cells to communicate properly[267] and in the construction of DNA.[268] Moreover, due to its connection with the immune system[269] and neurological problems, it is also included in the protocol.

For example, animal studies reveal that during pregnancy, adequate choline consumption is essential for the brain development of the fetus.[270] Moreover, **in studies using animal models of multiple sclerosis, choline promoted remyelination.**[271]

Myelin is the name given to a mixture of proteins and phospholipids forming a whitish insulating sheath around many nerve fibers, increasing the speed at which impulses are conducted. As previously mentioned, multiple sclerosis is caused by the attack of our immune cells against this insulating lining.

Imagine having a rat infestation in your home. In time, these mice end up gnawing at your TV's electrical cables. That's what our immune system does to our nerve fiber. Even if high-dose vitamin D therapy puts an end to this attack, our body still needs to correct what has been destroyed.

Rebuilding the myelin surrounding the nerve cells is therefore of vital importance. If choline is essential for the brain and the whole body and if there are studies demonstrating that, at least in animal models, it assists in this regenerative process then it makes perfect sense to recommend supplementing with choline, especially if you are fighting multiple sclerosis.

Magnesium

Dose recommended in the protocol: 125 to 250 milligrams of magnesium chloride or magnesium glycinate, 4 times per day.

Best taken: With food as it increases the absorption of magnesium.[272]

Daily total: Between 500 and 1,000 milligrams.

Magnesium is essential to life and is found in all living organisms.[273] In the human body, magnesium is involved in innumerable biological processes.[274] For this reason, the lack of magnesium is expected to cause many symptoms and problems.

At the same time, studies have shown that due to the depletion of our soils, the foods we consume have fewer and fewer minerals, such as magnesium.[275] In addition, magnesium undergoes several metabolic steps from being ingested all the way to being used by our body. Problems in any of these steps will eventually lead to symptoms of deficiency. That's how easy it is to get deficient. With what consequences?

A 2001 study[276] pointed out the diseases and problems associated with the insufficient magnesium, they include:

- Hypertension.
- Cardiovascular diseases.[277]
- Damage to the kidneys.
- Damage to the liver.
- Migraines.
- Multiple sclerosis.
- Glaucoma.
- Alzheimer's disease.
- Recurrent bacterial infections in the cavities — sinuses, vagina, ear, lung, throat, among others — due to low levels of nitric oxide.
- Yeast infections due to a depressed immune system.
- Low gastric acid and behavioral disorders due to a deactivation of thiamine.
- Premenstrual syndrome.

- Calcium deficiency, causing osteoporosis, hypertension, mood swings, among other problems.
- Dental caries.
- Loss of hearing.
- Type II diabetes.
- Cramps.
- Muscle weakness.
- Impotence due to a lack of nitrous oxide — studies have implicated arginine and pycnogenol as a possible solution for erectile dysfunction,[278] much in part due to the role of arginine in assisting the production of nitric oxide. Therefore, it makes sense that magnesium would be involved as well as it possesses an essential role in the production of nitric oxide.[279] Not to mention the association between vitamin D deficiency and erectile dysfunction.[280]
- Aggression, also related to the lack of nitric oxide.
- Fibroids.
- Potassium deficiency leading to arrhythmias and hypertension.
- Some forms of cancer.

In addition to all this, magnesium seems to be directly related to longevity because of the way **magnesium supplementation mimics the beneficial effects of caloric restriction.**[281, 282]

Hence the full potential of correcting a magnesium deficiency.

There are several forms of magnesium. Magnesium chloride is an excellent source because of the ease with which it can be purchased — and at a very low price, especially when compared to most supplements. Moreover, it has demonstrated some potential as an anticancer agent.[283] Buy it in bulk at your local pharmacy as "magnesium chloride hexahydrate."

Magnesium glycinate is also another good source of magnesium, but much more expensive.

Whichever source you choose, magnesium benefits are indisputable.

Vitamin B2

Recommended dose in the protocol: Between 50 to 100 milligrams, 4 times a day.
Best taken: With some food to reduce any gastric discomfort.
Daily total: Between 200 and 400 milligrams.

As noted in Chapter 5: "a study published by Dr. Coimbra and an associate in the *Brazilian Journal of Medical and Biological Research* had the following title: 'High doses of riboflavin and the elimination of dietary red meat promote the recovery of some motor functions in Parkinson's disease patients' [284]

In this article, the researchers refer to another study showing that in some populations, notably Florence and London, 10-15% of people have problems with the metabolism of riboflavin.[285] However, even those who don't have this metabolic issue can be deficient in riboflavin. For example, it is estimated that in Europe the riboflavin deficiency levels can reach up to 20%.[286]

Dr. Coimbra and his associate, Dr. Junqueira, solved the problem by administering between 24 and 30 milligrams of riboflavin per day.

Due to the prevalence of deficiencies resulting from a deficient metabolism of vitamin B2 and considering the important relationship between vitamin B2 and vitamin D, vitamin B2 is, along with magnesium, essential during the high-dose vitamin D protocol."

You will notice your body is metabolizing vitamin B2 because your urine will change color.[287]

Vitamin B12

Recommended dose in the protocol: Between 1,000 and 5,000 micrograms, 4 times a day.
Best taken: Away from meals, if using sublingual tablets.
Total daily: 5,000 to 20,000 micrograms.

As explained earlier in Appendix D: "Vitamin B12 is essential for the correct functioning of the nervous system. The lack of this essential vitamin causes dementia symptoms that can be confused with other better-known diseases such as Alzheimer's.

Vitamin B12 deficiency can get so serious as to cause psychotic problems and concentration deficits higher than those caused by Alzheimer's. However, vitamin B12 deficiency does not cause the pattern of language problems and apraxia characteristic of Alzheimer's disease. The apraxia is characterized by the inability to perform gestures as if all the brain machinery responsible for the execution of movements was damaged.

Dementia caused by insufficient vitamin B12 may be reversible with adequate vitamin B12 supplementation.[288] Dementia associated with Alzheimer's disease isn't curable, although high doses of vitamin D appear to have a connection with improved cognition[289] as well as supplementation with melatonin.[290]

However, dementia is one of the last symptoms of vitamin B12 deficiency. Being essential for the proper functioning of red blood cells, vitamin B12 deficiency causes a type of anemia called pernicious anemia, which leads to death unless the person receives adequate supplementation, usually through intramuscular injections.

In addition, the deficiency of this vitamin causes paresthesia, a type of pain that involves burn and electric shock sensations and tremors. These symptoms are like those caused by the destruction of the myelin sheets that occurs in multiple sclerosis.

In this regard, it's essential to ensure that vitamin B12 levels are well within the reference levels. This is especially important given the ease with which someone can become deficient. Just like with vitamin D, vitamin B12 absorption and metabolization involves many steps and these can be affected by the drugs you take or the quality of your digestive system and diet.

On diet, it's noteworthy that, in addition to cereals and other fortified foods, vitamin B12 is found mainly in animal products. Contrary to popular belief, however, vitamin B12 isn't unique to these foods, being also found in nori, in some algae and mushrooms, and in tempeh — a type of fermented soy.[291, 292]

In case of a deficiency, in addition to intramuscular injections, the patient may opt for oral supplementation. Here, I strongly recommend that methylcobalamin be chosen instead of cyanocobalamin. The difference between the two is like the difference between vitamin D3 and vitamin D2. Methylcobalamin requires fewer metabolization steps to become usable by our organism.

Vitamin B12 is directly related to folic acid. Both folic acid and vitamin B12 are included in the daily supplements recommended by Dr. Coimbra."

Most vitamin B12 supplements are in the form of a small tablet that is placed under the tongue until it melts — a sublingual tablet. But there are also transdermal patches and nasal sprays.

In most cases, you will opt for a sublingual tablet. Because of this, your vitamin B12 should be taken away from meals.

Folic Acid — Vitamin B9

Recommended dose in the protocol: 500 micrograms four times a day.
Best taken: With or without food.[293]
Total daily: 2,000 micrograms.

Folic acid is usually taken by a woman while she is pregnant. If the woman doesn't get sufficient levels of this vitamin the baby in her womb may develop serious health issues, such as heart problems and spina bifida[294] — a condition in which there's no closure of the neural tubes. In addition, folic acid helps the mother is too, who at risk of anemia and peripheral neuropathy.[295]

However, the importance of folic acid is not limited to a pregnant woman. Vitamin B9 is essential to life. Your immune system needs it[296] and without adequate levels, you may develop anemia,[297] and increase your risk of cardiovascular disease,[298, 299, 300] nervous system problems[301] and even Alzheimer's disease.[302] Folic acid deficiency is also directly related to an increased risk of cancer.[303, 304]

However, when supplementing with folic acid there is a problem you must be aware of. For our organism to make use of folic acid it first needs to convert it into a chemical called "L–5–methyltetrahydrofolate of calcium" — abbreviated 5–MTHF.[305] And as it turns out, many people have difficulties making this chemical conversion. Should you try and solve this problem by taking a higher amount of folic acid?

No. That would be a dangerous course of action. Why?

Because any folic acid that your organism fails to convert to 5–MTHF keeps accumulating in your body. This ends up being harmful.

Perhaps you are wondering: "So why not take 5–MTHF instead?"

This is indeed the best option. Folic acid is similar to vitamin D2 and cyanocobalamin — they are like the powder you need to add water to, stir and put in the microwave before you can eat the cake. 5–MTHF is like vitamin D3 and methylcobalamin — the cake is already ready to be eaten.

Studies have shown that our body absorbs 5–MTHF much better, especially if you are one of those whose body has difficulty converting folic acid to 5–MTHF.[306, 307]

Chromium Picolinate

Recommended protocol dose: 150 micrograms 4 times daily.

Best taken: 15 minutes before meals according to a small study[308] or according to the instructions on the label of the supplement.

Total daily: 600 micrograms.

As discussed earlier: "although chromium has been unanimously considered an essential mineral for decades,[309] in recent times its status of "essential mineral" has been called into question.[310] Despite this, this mineral has been shown to be pharmacologically active in certain animal clinical studies.[311] Even so, its ability to exert an effect on the human body has not yet gained unequivocal approval from the scientific community.[312]

Still, there are clinical studies demonstrating its positive effect on the human glucose metabolism.[313, 314] For example, in *Clinical studies on chromium picolinate supplementation in diabetes mellitus – a review*, the conclusion of the researchers, after reviewing 15 studies, was as follows:

"All 15 studies showed salutary effects in at least one parameter of diabetes management, including dyslipidemia. Positive outcomes from [chromium picolinate] supplementation included reduced blood glucose, insulin, cholesterol, and triglyceride levels and reduced requirements for hypoglycemic medication." And: "The pooled data from studies using [chromium picolinate] supplementation for type 2 diabetes mellitus subjects show substantial reductions in hyperglycemia and hyperinsulinemia, which equate to a reduced risk for disease complications. Collectively, the data support the safety and therapeutic value of [chromium picolinate] for the management of cholesterolemia and hyperglycemia in subjects with diabetes."[315]

It is clear why chromium picolinate is recommended by Dr. Coimbra in its protocol, even amongst the controversy within the scientific community as to whether chromium is an essential mineral.

However, because of the toxic potential of this substance when in excess, it makes sense to keep tight control over its blood levels.

This is especially important given how chromium toxicity manifests itself in renal function.[316]

As noted, the kidneys are our greatest ally against excess calcium in the blood. We want our kidneys to maintain their filtering and excretory capacities at the highest possible level. Therefore, if you are taking chromium picolinate it is essential to keep up to date on the levels of this mineral in your blood."

Selenium

Recommended dose in the protocol: Between 50 and 100 micrograms, 4 times per day.

Best taken: With a meal to reduce the chances of stomach cramps.

Daily total: Between 200 and 400 micrograms.

Selenium is an essential mineral, vital for the proper functioning of the human body. However, it is a mineral that we need in small amounts. Think micrograms instead of milligrams.

Even so, these micrograms work wonders. Selenium is essential for brain function and is helpful in fighting brain cancer.[317] It is vital for the proper functioning of our immune system,[318, 319] making, as an example, the influenza virus less aggressive to the lungs[320] and even improving white blood cell count in patients with HIV[321] all the while delaying the progress of HIV to AIDS.[322] In addition, it has an immunomodulatory effect, reducing inflammation.[323, 324]

Selenium deficiency is related to heart disease,[325] neuromuscular disorders,[326] cancer[327, 328] and male infertility.[329]

Selenium is essential for the adequate functioning of the thyroid,[330] and has shown potential, still under investigation,[331] in the case of Hashimoto's when taken together with iodine.[332]

Hashimoto's is an autoimmune disorder in which the thyroid becomes the target of the immune system. Moreover, due to the similarity of some structures in our eye with the thyroid cells being targeted, the immune system ends up attacking the eyes, especially in patients with a thyroid pathology called Graves' disease.

You may have this health issue yourself, or you may have noticed that some people with thyroid disease also have protruding eyes. There is a study describing how selenium has a beneficial effect on this condition, according to the bibliographical note.[333]

However, taking selenium in amounts higher than those recommended by Dr. Coimbra can be dangerous. Selenium is a mineral that is toxic in high doses and may cause adverse effects. There is at least one report of a death related to excess selenium supplementation.[334] In the case described, a 75-year-old man ingested 10 grams of selenium in the form of sodium selenite to treat prostate cancer. The man died a few hours later from cardiac arrest.

However, 10 grams correspond to 10,000,000 — ten million micrograms. This dose is 25,000 times higher than the maximum daily dose of 400 micrograms you would be taking in the protocol.

This means you don't need to be afraid to take selenium at the recommended doses, quite the opposite.

Researchers in Beijing, China, investigated older populations. The study included 208 centenarians and 238 people in their 90s. They discovered something very interesting: In these centenarians, the levels of some minerals, like selenium, were higher than normal.[335] It seems selenium, in the correct dose, does not kill, quite the opposite.

Also, in a study lasting 9 years, researchers at the University of Montpellier in conjunction with colleagues at the La Colombière Hospital in France found that the blood levels of selenium were inversely related to the likelihood of someone dying.

Those who had the lowest levels of selenium at the start of the study had a 54% greater chance of dying than those with the highest levels. In turn, the risk of dying specifically from cancer was assessed as being 79% higher in this group of people with low levels of selenium.[336, 337]

What is the conclusion? If you want to increase your chances of living longer ensure that your selenium levels are adequate.

How should you supplement selenium?

There are several forms of selenium. Sodium selenite is just one of the kinds of selenium supplements available, with several online forums describing experimental anticancer protocols involving high doses of this form of selenium.

There is also selenium sourced from yeasts. One of these yeasts, called *saccharomyces cerevisiae*, also known as brewer's yeast, is placed in an environment rich in sodium selenite. This causes the yeast to absorb the selenium and process it, producing a chemical compound containing a type of selenium that is more bioavailable to humans.[338] This type of selenium was used in the many of studies mentioned in this book. This form of selenium has also been shown to be safe even when taken at a dose of 800 micrograms, daily, for several years.[339]

But maybe the simplest form of selenium is already in your house.

One study stated that the amount of selenium present in a Brazil nut can reach up to 30 micrograms.[340] That means if you eat 7 nuts a day you have the potential to be ingesting 210 micrograms of selenium! I say "potential" because the final amount of selenium present in the nuts you are eating depends on several factors, including the quality of the soil on which the nut was grown.

Another study is even more impressive, demonstrating that Brazil nuts selenium content can reach up to 159 micrograms.[341] In that case, three of these nuts would give you 477 micrograms of selenium, more than the maximum daily dose of 400 micrograms you'd get on the Coimbra protocol. In turn, a Brazil nut, native to the Brazilian state of Mato Grosso, may contain only 7 micrograms. These being the only Brazilian states mentioned in the quoted study.

And what about the effect of Brazil nuts on cholesterol?

Researchers from Santa Maria, Rio Grande do Sul, Brazil, carried out a study with ten people between the ages of 23 and 34.[342]

Although total cholesterol levels did not change, the researchers observed a significant drop in LDL levels — the so-called "bad" cholesterol — and an equally impressive increase in "good" cholesterol — HDL. Even more impressive is the fact that this positive effect was maintained even after 30 days.

This positive effect was observed after they consumed either 20 grams or 50 grams of Brazil nuts. If we consider that each nut weights about 5 grams, this means that consuming 4 to 10 nuts **on a single occasion** has the potential to lower and **keep your cholesterol low for at least 30 days.**

These images, made available in the clinical study, are worth a thousand words:

- "Bad" cholesterol:

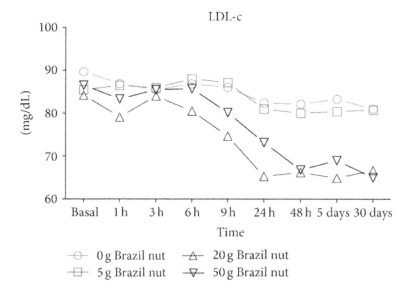

- "Good" cholesterol:

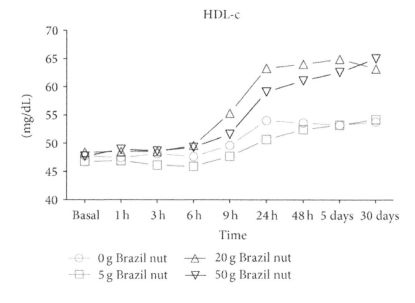

These results lead the researchers to conclude: "Interestingly, the ingestion of 20 g of Brazil nut determined a more pronounced decrease in LDL-c levels as well as a higher increase in HDL-c than did 50 g. These results suggest that **eating an average of 4 nuts might be enough to improve the levels of LDL-c and HDL-c for up to 30 days.**" — emphasis added.

And of course, if the goal is cholesterol reduction there are other supplements, such as pantethine,[343] a precursor of vitamin B5.

Coenzyme Q10 (Coq10)

Recommended protocol dose: 100 micrograms per day, optionally.

Best taken: With meals. First, because some of the supplements containing Coq10, provide you with a form that is fat soluble (meaning it needs to be ingested with some fat). Secondly, because Coq10 is absorbed in your intestine, hence, a slower intestinal transit, derived from the ingestion of the molecule along with food, will result in a superior absorption.[344]

Daily total: 100 micrograms.

A cell is like a city, and just as a city needs energy, so does the cell.

In cities, energy is produced in power plants. In our cells, energy is produced in the mitochondria. How?

When we breathe and eat we are putting energy in the form of oxygen, fat and glucose inside our bodies. These components are carried by our blood to each of our cells. After entering the cell, they are taken to the mitochondria where they are transformed into ATP — the fuel of our body.

This transformation generates waste in the form of water and carbon dioxide. These waste materials are then expelled through the urine and respiration in the case of water and only through respiration in the case of carbon dioxide. This process is similar to the way a car's exhaust system disposes of the gases resulting from the engine's combustion.

What is the role of coenzyme Q10 in all this?

Coenzyme Q10 is essential for our mitochondria.

Imagine what would happen to your car if you removed the battery. You would turn the key, and nothing would happen, even though the engine was intact, and the tank had fuel. Likewise, without coenzyme Q10 the mitochondria won't work — not even you try to push it!

Coenzyme Q10 is especially important for our heart cells[345] and there is a direct relationship between the degree of coenzyme Q10 deficiency and the severity of heart disease.[346]

If our heart beats on average 70 times a minute that's over 100,000 beats per day. This means that our heart cells require a lot of energy. Their mitochondria are always working, always depending on coenzyme Q10 to produce energy efficiently.[347]

In addition, coenzyme Q10 has another important function.

When our mitochondria produce energy they also produce the so-called free radicals. Again, the illustration of the car engine will help us take the point home. When fuel enters the engine, it is ignited by an electric spark, which causes an explosion. This explosion pushes a part of the engine called a piston.

As you may imagine, all these explosions stress the engine.

Therefore, an engine must be built with quality materials, capable of enduring all those blasts for years on end. Similarly, when the mitochondria produce energy this also causes stress in the form of particles called free radicals.

These free radicals need to be neutralized or they'll damage the entire cellular structure.[348] Coenzyme Q10 plays a key role in this by acting as an antioxidant.[349] Due to all these vital functions it's no wonder that coenzyme Q10 is directly linked to our well-being and health.

Thus, a number of clinical studies[350] have shown a link between coenzyme Q10 levels and cardiovascular disease.[351, 352, 353, 354, 355, 356] Coenzyme Q10 deficiency may even be one reason why some people won't respond to their heart medication.[357] In addition, a relationship has been found between coenzyme Q10 and many different health issues, including cancer,[358] neurodegenerative [359, 360, 361, 362, 363] and ocular diseases[364] such as glaucoma,[365] diabetes,[366] among many other health problems related to oxidative stress.[367]

Among the list of beneficial effects of this coenzyme is also the protection against the toxic effects of cyclosporine over the kidneys,[368] an immunosuppressant drug used to prevent the body from rejecting transplanted organs.

Thus, supplementation with coenzyme Q10 is especially important for the person who has heart or neurodegenerative problems.

When it comes time to choose a supplement, we come across two options. Ubiquinol[369] and ubiquinone. What is the difference?

Supplements containing the active form — ubiquinol — are more expensive but more active in our body.[370] Supplements containing ubiquinone are cheaper but more difficult to absorb, ultimately resulting in inferior results when compared to ubiquinol.[371]

The manufacturers of supplements try to play with the ignorance of the general public. For example, if you look for "Coenzyme Q10" you will find bottles with labels that *only* say "Coenzyme Q10" or "Coq10." Usually, these contain ubiquinone, the weakest form.

Don't let yourself be fooled by clever marketing.

Bottles containing ubiquinol will make this clear to you on the label. They are more expensive than ubiquinone, but if you have a heart problem they are a better option. Of course, if your budget just allows you to make use of the cheaper form, ubiquinone, this is better than nothing.

Appendix F

High-Dose Vitamin D Protocol — The Summary

What's our goal?

- **To increase vitamin D levels to the maximum extent possible.** This will give your body the best chances of dealing with the health problems you are facing.

  If you have an autoimmune disease this will mean boosting vitamin D until the immune system is forced to react by stopping its attack against its host — you.

How do we know we've reached our goal?

- We have reached our goal when (1) **PTH levels are at the lower end of the reference range** and (2) **any additional reason for a low PTH has been ruled out**, such as (2.1) high calcium levels or (2.2) pre-existing hypoparathyroidism.

How should we adjust the amount of vitamin D we are taking?

- If PTH is not yet at the minimum value allowed by the laboratory reference range, the daily dose of vitamin D should be increased by 10,000 or 20,000 IU and maintained at that new level until the next blood tests results.

- If PTH is below the minimum value the dose of vitamin D should be reduced.

- If calcium is above the reference values, vitamin D may be reduced or stopped for a few days. Increased attention should be paid to calcium and fluid intake and renal function needs to be monitored even closer.

  You can continue with a lower dosage or with the same

dosage if it turns out that the problem was the diet rather than the kidneys.

These adjustments should be made in line with laboratory results and under proper medical supervision to exclude kidney problems as the root cause of the higher than normal calcium levels.

What special steps should we take as vitamin D dosages increase?

- It is imperative to **reduce calcium-rich foods intake**. For at least three reasons:

    1. High doses of vitamin D promote high intestinal calcium absorption and higher bone demineralization.

    2. High levels of calcium cause a reduction in PTH levels, which can give us the false impression that we are already taking the correct dose of vitamin D.

    3. In an attempt to keep calcium levels under control, the kidneys may become overloaded and if there's an insufficient fluid intake kidney stones may form.

- It is vital to **drink plenty of water** — 2.5 liters (2.64 quarts) of fluids a day, including juices, teas and other sources — as this will help the kidneys by decreasing mineral concentration in the renal filtration channels.

- Take care of your kidneys by drinking **"Herbensurina" type teas**,[372] as prescribed by Dr. Manuel Pinto Coelho, who we recall, reports that he has yet to find a case of vitamin D induced hypercalcemia in his clinical practice — or an equivalent tea available in your area since this formulation is from a laboratory based in Spain, in Europe. Thus, for your reference while in the search for a similar tea, Herbensurina tea is composed of:

1. Herniaria Glabra (*Herniaria glabra L.*) (Whole plant) 1 gram per sachet.

2. *Agropyron repens (L.) P. Beauv.* (rhizome) 0.25 grams per sachet.

3. Horsetail (*Equisetum arvense L.*) (sterile stems) 0.15 grams per sachet.

4. Elderflower (*Sambucus nigra L.*) (flowers) 0.1 grams per sachet.

- You can't lead a sedentary life. A sedentary lifestyle will not stimulate your bones to reabsorb calcium, which will cause an unnecessary loss of bone density. It is therefore essential to **exercise** and to **walk**. If your doctor agrees, you can take a **bone densitometry test**, repeated at the end of each year in the protocol, to ensure that your bone density stays within a healthy range.

- **Vitamin K2** is an extra helper. It stimulates your bones to absorb calcium and should be taken at least at a dose of 100 micrograms per 10,000 IU of vitamin D. The independent investigator Jeff T. Bowles recommends 200 mcg of vitamin K2 MK-7 with 1,000 mcg of vitamin K2 MK-4 per 10,000 IU of vitamin D.

- You should **be aware of the symptoms of hypercalcemia**. Hypercalcemia should be treated with a total or partial reduction of vitamin D supplementation, or even bisphosphonates — administered under qualified medical supervision.

- Proper medical follow-up and regular **blood and urine tests** are of equal importance. At the very least you should be regularly testing:

  1. **Vitamin D.** To access your risk hypercalcemia risk, especially after your levels rise to 100 ng/mL or higher.

  2. **PTH.** Fundamental to understanding if your body is reacting to vitamin D or not.

  3. **Blood calcium (total and ionized).** Vital to ensure that you aren't at risk for hypercalcemia and to cross-reference with the PTH result to check for any signs of hypoparathyroidism (low calcium and low PTH) or hyperparathyroidism (high calcium and high PTH). Also, knowledge of your calcium levels will allow you to evaluate if a low PTH result is a potential false positive or not.

  4. **24-hour urine calcium.** Essential for checking the state of your kidneys and your potential for developing kidney stones.

- *Ideally*, we will do **regular tests** — every 2 months according to some doctors or even every six months in Dr. Coimbra's protocol — **to more than 20 parameters** that will ensure that all key organs and metabolites are within the expected range — as defined in Chapter 5, and in greater detail in Appendix D.

- Take **extra supplements**, in addition to vitamin K2, including at a minimum:

  1. **Vitamin B2** (50 to 100 milligrams, 4 times per day).
  2. **Magnesium chloride** (125 to 250 milligrams, 4 times per day).

- In *ideal* situations, where your budget allows, we will include each of the **supplements** listed in Chapter 5, within the dosages recommended there.

- Talk to your doctor if you are taking any drugs that may influence coagulation, such as anticoagulants or the pill, due to vitamin K2 and its potential to be converted into vitamin K1.

- Talk to your doctor if you are taking any drugs that affect the metabolism of vitamin D, such as antacids, cortisone and its derivatives or any of the nephrotoxic drugs listed in Appendix G. Whenever possible look for alternative drugs without these side effects — if they are available.

Appendix G

59 Drugs That Can Hurt Your Kidneys and Ruin Your Chances of Staying on The Protocol

Accarding to a study published in the *Journal of Renal Injury Prevention* in 2015,[373] the most common toxic drugs for the kidneys are:

Medication	Drug category	Renal toxicity
Acetaminophen	Non-narcotic analgesic	Chronic interstitial nephritis, acute tubular necrosis
Acetazolamide	Carbonic-anhydrase inhibitor	Proximal renal tubular acidosis
Acyclovir	Antiviral	Acute interstitial nephritis, crystal nephropathy
Allopurinol	Hypouricemic agent	Acute interstitial nephritis
Aspirin	Non-narcotic analgesic	Chronic interstitial nephritis
Amitriptyline	Antidepressant	Rhabdomyolysis
Aminoglycosides	Antimicrobial	Acute tubular necrosis
Amphotericin B	Antifungal	Acute tubular necrosis, distal renal tubular acidosis
Angiotensin-converting enzyme inhibitors (ACEI)	Antihypertensive	Acute kidney injury
Angiotensin receptor blockers (ARB)	Antihypertensive	Acute kidney injury
Benzodiazepines	Sedative-Hypnotic	Rhabdomyolysis
Beta lactams	Antimicrobial	Acute interstitial nephritis
Carbenicillin	Antimicrobial	Metabolic alkalosis
Cephalosporin	Antimicrobial	Acute tubular necrosis

Chlorpropamide	Sulfonylureas	Hyponatremia, syndrome inappropriate ADH secretion
Cimetidine	Gastrointestinal	Acute interstitial nephritis
Cisplatin	Antineoplastic	Chronic interstitial nephritis
Clopidogrel	Antiplatelet	Thrombotic microangiopathy
Cocaine	Narcotic analgesic	Rhabdomyolysis
Contrast agents	Contrast medium	Acute tubular necrosis
Cortisone	Corticosteroid	Metabolic alkalosis, hypertension
Cyclophosphamide	Antineoplastic	Hemorrhagic cystitis
Cyclosporine	Immunosuppressive	Acute tubular necrosis, chronic interstitial nephritis, thrombotic microangiopathy
D-penicillamine	Antirheumatic	Nephrotic syndrome
Diphenhydramine	Antihistamine	Rhabdomyolysis
Furosemide	Loop diuretic	Acute interstitial nephritis
Ganciclovir	Antiviral	Crystal nephropathy
Gold Na thiomalate	Antiarthritic	Glomerulonephritis, nephrotic syndrome
Haloperidol	Antipsychotic	Rhabdomyolysis
Indinavir	Antiviral	Acute interstitial nephritis, crystal nephropathy
Interferon-alfa	Antineoplastic	Glomerulonephritis
Lansoprazole	Proton pump inhibitor	Acute interstitial nephritis
Lithium	Antipsychotic	Chronic interstitial nephritis, glomerulonephritis, rhabdomyolysis

Methadone	Narcotic analgesic	Rhabdomyolysis
Methamphetamine	Psychostimulant	Rhabdomyolysis
Methotrexate	Antineoplastic	Crystal nephropathy
Mitomycin-C	Antineoplastic	Thrombotic microangiopathy
Naproxen	Nonsteroidal anti-inflammatory	Acute and chronic interstitial nephritis, acute tubular necrosis, glomerulonephritis
Omeprazole	Proton pump inhibitor	Acute interstitial nephritis
Pamidronate acid	Bisphosphonate, osteoporosis prevention	Glomerulonephritis
Pantoprazole	Proton pump inhibitor	Acute interstitial nephritis
Penicillin G	penicillin	Glomerulonephritis
Pentamidine	Antimicrobial	Acute tubular necrosis
Phenformin	Hypoglycemic	Lactic acidosis
Phenacetin	Non-narcotic analgesic	Chronic interstitial nephritis
Phenytoin	Anticonvulsant	Acute interstitial nephritis, diabetes insipidus
Probenecid	Uricosuric	Crystal nephropathy, nephrotic syndrome
Puromycin	Antimicrobial	Nephrotic syndrome
Quinine	Muscle relaxant	Thrombotic microangiopathic
Quinolones	Antimicrobial	Acute interstitial nephritis, crystal nephropathy

Rifampin	Antimicrobial	Acute interstitial nephritis
Ranitidine	Gastrointestinal	Acute interstitial nephritis
Statins	Lipid-lowering	Rhabdomyolysis
Sulfonamides	Antimicrobial	Acute interstitial nephritis, crystal nephropathy
Tacrolimus	Immunosuppressive	Acute tubular necrosis
Tetracycline	Antimicrobial	Acute tubular necrosis
Azides	Diuretic	Acute interstitial nephritis
Tolbutamide	Hypoglycemic	Nephrotic syndrome
Vancomycin	Antimicrobial	Acute interstitial nephritis

Are you taking any of these medications?

If it has been prescribed by your doctor and is a drug that you must take every day talk to him about the possibility of replacing it with a drug that is less toxic to the kidneys. If this isn't possible, be sure to be even more zealous about liquid ingestion to try and keep the drug concentrations in your kidneys as small as possible. More water being ingested equals fewer drug molecules per volume of liquid moving across your kidneys.

If the drug has not been prescribed, such as acetaminophen, talk to your pharmacist about an alternative that does not harm your kidneys as much.

Remember: It is dangerous to stop taking a drug that has been prescribed by your doctor for a specific illness. This does not mean that you should take everything that is blindly prescribed to you. Why? Because taking medications is one of the leading causes of death in the United States. Half of these deaths are the result of taking drugs *as prescribed by the doctor*.[374] So try to be balanced and talk to your doctor about what drugs you *really* need to be taking.

Once you feel better, ask the doctor to adjust your dose accordingly.

Appendix H

Do You Remember?

A s promised in the introduction, this final Appendix contains a compilation of all the "Do you remember?" sections and its purpose is twofold.

First, it is very useful to be able to quickly review and recall the most important concepts in the book. This means you won't need to reread the entire book to find the key points. Secondly, this Appendix gives you a quick outline you can use as the basis for a conversation with a doctor or with another person interested in learning more about vitamin D, vitamin K2 and the experimental protocols.

Happy recap!

Introduction

Questions:

A. Is vitamin D, a vitamin or a hormone?

B. In a nutshell, what is a hormone?

C. A hormone has the same effect in all the cells receiving it? Give an example.

D. Why is Vitamin D often called the super hormone?

Answers:

A. Vitamin D, in its active form, is actually a hormone and not a vitamin.

B. A hormone is a molecule the body uses to send messages to its cells.

C. Each cell reacts to each hormone differently, depending on the instructions stored in our genetic code, or DNA.

   For example, adrenaline is a hormone that stimulates the lungs and the heart while concurrently instructing the stomach cells to stop producing protective mucus.

D. Vitamin D is considered a super hormone because it seems to positively affect the entire human body.

Chapter 1

No, Vitamin D is Not Harmless

Questions:

A. What is the function of the parathyroid glands?

B. What is the role of PTH?

C. Besides the parathyroid glands, which other organ helps with calcium regulation?

D. How does vitamin D influence calcium absorption in the small intestine?

E. What is the effect of a high dose of vitamin D on bone tissue?

F. What are the dangers associated with Vitamin D supplementation?

On the next page you will find the answers.

Answers:

A. The parathyroid glands protect us from low blood levels of calcium by producing more PTH in response to a drop in calcium levels. By contrast, when calcium levels increase they produce less PTH.

B. PTH is a hormone with a double function: it stimulates bone tissues to release more calcium while concurrently stimulating the kidneys to activate more vitamin D.

C. The kidneys.

D. Vitamin D stimulates the intestine to absorb more calcium from foods.

E. High doses of vitamin D further stimulate bone calcium release.

F. Taking high doses of vitamin D on a continuous basis may cause blood calcium levels to rise too much, causing hypercalcemia to develop.

Chapter 2

Why Supplement with High Vitamin D Doses?

Questions:

A. Despite the enormous technological advances in diagnostics, what problem remains in the field of neurology?

B. Why are most doctors unaware of the latest clinical findings related to the use of high-dose vitamin D therapy?

C. What were the findings some doctors uncovered as they engaged in more detailed research on the therapeutic value of vitamin D?

D. What's Dr. Coimbra success rate with patients suffering from Multiple Sclerosis?

Answers:

A. Existing official treatment options help relieve symptoms and make the diseases progress more slowly. Yet, most of the times, they don't offer much hope beyond that.

B. Because these studies haven't gained worldwide attention and approval within the medical ecosystem.

C. Some doctors who dug deep into scientific databases found a clear pattern revealing the therapeutic potential of vitamin D in autoimmune disease processes.

D. 95% go into complete remission, 5% report improvement but not complete remission.

Chapter 3

Why Isn't high-dose vitamin D Common Medical Practice Yet?

Questions:

A. Why can we say a disease is an emergent process?

B. How can we cure any disease?

C. What is the problem with many promising clinical trials?

D. Why does it take so long for a doctor to start prescribing a treatment that has shown promise in the treatment of humans?

E. Why isn't the use of high doses of vitamin D a common medical practice?

Answers:

A. A disease is an emergent process because it can only continue for as long as all the factors contributing to its development remain present.

B. To cure any disease, we "only" need to discover how to influence enough parts of the processes contributing to its maintenance.

C. The problem with many promising studies is that the results obtained in laboratory tests involving animals don't translate to humans in the same way.

D. A physician is trained to follow pre-established protocols. Doing so protects them from criminal prosecution.

E. The use of high doses of vitamin D isn't a common medical practice because there aren't enough clinical studies to satisfy all the requirements of the medical community, like double-blind, placebo-controlled trials. For these reasons, high-dose vitamin D therapy isn't part of the official medical protocols yet.

Chapter 4

Dispelling the Confusion Between D2, D3, Micrograms and International Units

Questions:

A. What is the difference between Vitamin D2 and Vitamin D3?

B. 1 IU of vitamin D is equivalent to how many micrograms?

C. 1 Microgram of Vitamin D equals how many IU?

D. In the United States, what is the recommended daily allowance set for vitamin D?

E. What is the commonality between autoimmune diseases and what sets them apart?

F. What is the basic logic behind high–dose vitamin D therapy?

Answers:

A. Vitamin D2 must be further transformed into vitamin D3 before being used by the body. This extra step means the body has more difficulty using vitamin D2 than vitamin D3.

B. 1 IU of vitamin D is equivalent to 0.025 mcg.

C. 1 mcg of vitamin D is equivalent to 40 IU.

D. The recommended daily allowance in the United States is 600 IU (15 mcg) for an adult aged 70 or younger, and 800 IU (20 mcg) for anyone older.

E. All autoimmune diseases are caused by an immune system gone mad. The difference is in the tissue or organ being attacked.

F. In high-dose vitamin D therapy, the dosage is gradually increased until the blood concentration of vitamin D is sufficiently high to exert control over the immune system.

Chapter 5

How to Supplement
High Doses of Vitamin D Safely?

Questions:

A.   What is the safe vitamin D upper limit according to most vitamin D experts?

B.   What are the 6 steps to sunbathe safely and effectively?

C.   What are the 6 steps to supplement vitamin D safely and effectively?

D.   What is the vitamin D starting dose used in experimental protocols?

E.   What is the variation in the dose of vitamin K2 used in experimental protocols?

Answers:

A. The general accepted vitamin D upper limit among vitamin D experts is 10,000 IU — 250 micrograms.

B. The six steps to sunbathe safely and effectively are: (1) Going out into the sun. Afterall, glass blocks UVB. (2) Choosing the best time interval, between 11:00 am and 3:00 pm. (3) Don't cover your entire body with clothes. Clothes block UVB radiation just like glass does. (4) Don't wear sunscreen. (5) Sunbath for just long enough for your skin to start turning pink. As a general rule of thumb this means sunbathing for half the time it would take sunlight to burn your skin. (6) Take a bath only a few hours after sun exposure.

C. The six steps to supplement vitamin D safely and effectively are: (1) Start with 10,000 IU per day. (2) Test your kidneys by measuring 24-hour urinary calcium and checking your blood levels of calcium, PTH and vitamin D with the 25(OH)D or 25-hydroxycholecalciferol test. (3) Understand the goal isn't just to increase vitamin D blood levels. Your focus is lowering blood PTH levels to the minimum allowed by the reference range. (4) Reduce consumption of calcium, increase the consumption of water and seek to lead a physically active life without too much stress. (5) Supplement at least with vitamin K2, vitamin B2 and magnesium chloride. (6) Repeat the blood tests periodically and adjust your vitamin D and vitamin K2 doses accordingly.

D. The base dosage used on experimental protocols is 1,000 IU of vitamin D per kilogram of body weight (1,000 IU per 2.20 pounds). This dosing is then either increased or decreased according to lab results.

E. The common dose of vitamin K2 used is of 100 mcg per 10,000 IU of vitamin D. Although in some cases it can get much higher. The independent researcher Jeff T. Bowles recommends 200 mcg of vitamin K2 MK-7 taken together with 1,000 mcg of vitamin K2 MK-4 per 10,000 IU of vitamin D.

Chapter 6

Vitamin D and the Immune System
— the science behind high-dose therapy

Questions:

A. What is inflammation?

B. What are the positive aspects of the inflammatory response?

C. What are the negative aspects of the inflammatory response?

D. How do immunosuppressants drugs work?

E. What is the name of the white blood cell responsible for stopping the inflammatory response?

F. How does vitamin D differ from immunosuppressants in its mechanism of action?

Answers:

A. When it detects an intruder or a cell of the body that needs to be destroyed — like a cancer cell — the immune system produces chemicals aimed at destroying the enemy while at the same time stimulating the body to send more blood and fluids to the area.

B. The extra blood and fluids reaching the affected area carry with them nutrients and platelets, which promotes healing, and more immune cells. In addition, extra fluids serve as a blockade against the propagation of intruders.

C. Inflammatory cytokines and other chemicals released during an extended inflammatory response cause irritation and damage to the surrounding healthy tissues.

D. Immunosuppressant drugs attempt to interrupt the chain of events that leads to the activation of a full-blown inflammatory response.

E. The white blood cell responsible for stopping the inflammatory response is called regulatory T cell.

F. Vitamin D enhances the communication within the immune system and promotes the production of regulatory T cells.

Chapter 7

Vitamin K2 — Making Friends With The Unknown Healer

Questions:

A.   What is the function of vitamin K1?

B.   What is the relationship between vitamin K1 and calcium?

C.   What is the function of vitamin K2?

D.   What is the relationship between vitamin K2 and calcium?

E.   What is the difference between vitamin K2 MK-4 and vitamin K2 MK-7?

Answers:

A. Vitamin K1 is an essential molecule in the blood clotting cascade. It has a format that fits the clotting factors and modifies them to allow them to attach to calcium. It's as if vitamin K were a master key, and each of the coagulation factors had a lock requiring vitamin K to come in to unlock some of their functions.

B. Vitamin K1 activates the calcium binding property of coagulation factors. Without the action of vitamin K1, coagulation factors would be unable to remain on the surface of the phospholipid table.

C. Vitamin K2 is responsible for activating osteocalcin and MGP, allowing them to interact with calcium.

D. Osteocalcin is present in bones and teeth and MGP is present in soft tissues. When vitamin K2 activates MGP, this causes calcium to leave our soft tissues. When vitamin K2 activates osteocalcin, this causes calcium to bind to our bones. Thus, vitamin K2 acts as a calcium carrier of sorts, removing calcium from where it shouldn't be and taking it to where it's needed.

E. The difference is in the source and format of the molecule. Vitamin K2 MK-4 is found mainly in animal products. Vitamin K2 MK-7 is found in foods that suffered bacterial fermentation. Due to their differences in format, vitamin K2 MK-7 is better absorbed and stays detectable in the human body for longer periods of time.

Chapter 8

Is Vitamin D
Superior to Antidepressants?

Questions:

A.   What is the stress response?

B.   What is the relationship between depression and...
     a.   ...adrenaline?
     b.   ...serotonin?
     c.   ...norepinephrine?
     d.   ...dopamine?
     e.   ...vitamin D?

C.   What were the vitamin D doses used in clinical studies and with what result?

Answers:

A. The stress response is an emergency mode designed to transform our body into a fleeing or fighting machine, a sort of superhuman mode. Several hormones and neurotransmitters work together so that our bodies place any non-essential processes in standby, while at the same time prioritizing survival related mechanisms.

B. The relationships are as follows:

    a. Adrenaline is one of the hormones responsible for the activation of the stress response. Under the effect of adrenaline, our heart beats faster, our breathing rate increases, and nutrient-rich blood and oxygen are diverted from the stomach, and other momentarily non-essential organs, towards the muscles to increase our chances of survival. If the stress response remains active for too long it will cause the depletion of our body's resources and deregulate serotonin, dopamine and norepinephrine levels, causing a negative effect felt strongly on the brain.

    b. Serotonin controls our ability to obsess on a subject. Low levels make us get caught in a subject. High levels help us relax. In depression, serotonin drops, making it difficult for us to stop thinking about our problems.

    c. Norepinephrine is essential for the proper functioning of the nervous system. When its levels drop, thinking and moving becomes harder. A point may come where simple movements seem colossal tasks. Low enough norepinephrine levels are responsible for the onset of psychomotor retardation. Really low levels of this key chemical can render a person unable to get out of bed. All these are typical symptoms of deep depression.

    d. Dopamine is the chemical of pleasure. When a person enters a state of depression he will have a hard time feeling any pleasure, this is because the metabolism of dopamine is affected by the underlying root causes of depression.

e. Vitamin D can modify the whole axis of organs and glands responsible for the activation and management of the stress response and of our hormones and neurotransmitters. Thus, vitamin D plays a fundamental role in the development and treatment of depression.

C. In clinical studies, doses of vitamin D varied between 400 and 18,400 IU. The results observed showed that vitamin D had at least the same effect as antidepressants — without the side effects.

Chapter 9

Vitamin D and Autism

Questions:

A. What is autism?

B. What is Asperger's syndrome?

C. What is the relationship between vitamin D and autism?

Answers:

A. Autism is a disorder affecting the development of the nervous system, including the brain, where several areas, notably those related to socio-emotional processing, don't develop in a typical way. This atypical development manifests itself in the form of atypical behaviors and attitudes. Autism exists on a spectrum, meaning that one can be more or less autistic depending on the severity of their difficulties processing socio-emotional information, among other behavioral and psychological factors.

B. Asperger's syndrome is a mild form of autism, characterized by a brain with difficulties processing nonverbal information. Someone with Asperger's syndrome can be mistakenly assumed to be arrogant or uninterested in others and their feelings.

C. Recent clinical studies have shown that supplementation with vitamin D can reduce the symptoms of autism. Also, recent research shows that if this supplementation is provided to the woman while she is still pregnant, the chances of her child being born with autism decreases.

Chapter 10

Vitamin D and Vitamin K2 Against Cancer

Questions:

A. What are the 10 key hallmarks of a cancer cell?

B. Why do vitamin D and vitamin K2 have such a significant effect on a person's chances of getting cancer?

Answers:

A.   A cancer cell has 10 key characteristics:

> a. the development of the capacity to allow itself to divide;
>
> b. the ability to ignore external instructions to stop dividing;
>
> c. the loss of the ability to self-destruct;
>
> d. the development of the capacity to exceed its own multiplication limit;
>
> e. the development of the ability to convince the body to give it more nourishment by means of angiogenesis;
>
> f. the acquisition of the ability to abandon the tumor site and enter the bloodstream;
>
> g. the ability to convince the immune system to help the cancer cells in their growth efforts;
>
> h. the development of the ability to pretend to be a healthy cell;
>
> i. genomic instability, that is, constant genetic mutation;
>
> j. the dependence on the fermentation of glucose as a source of cellular energy, which in turn provides the cancer cell with the necessary raw material to build new versions of itself.
>
> Although all these 10 characteristics may not be

present, if the cancer is left untreated, all of them will have the tendency to manifest.

B. Both vitamin D and vitamin K2 affect several of the characteristics that define a cell as cancerous. In addition, they achieve this in a synergistic manner, by exerting their effect in different ways.

Chapter 11

Heart Disease, Osteoporosis and Autoimmunity Were Just the Beginning: Asthma, Type 1 and Type 2 Diabetes, the Flu, Cold, Fibromyalgia, and Chronic Pain — No Stone Is Left Unturned

Questions:

A.   What is asthma?

B.   What is the relationship between vitamin D and asthma?

C.   What is type 1 diabetes?

D.   What is the relationship between vitamin D and type 1 diabetes?

E.   What is type 2 diabetes?

F.   What is the relationship between vitamin D and type 2 diabetes?

G.   What is the relationship between vitamin D and respiratory tract infections?

H.   What is the relationship between vitamin D and fibromyalgia and other diseases involving chronic pain of unknown origin?

Answers:

A.   Asthma is the chronic inflammation of our airways along with a tissue hypersensitivity to invading particles and microorganisms.

B.   Vitamin D promotes a reduction of symptoms. This is because it acts as an immunomodulator, decreasing tissue hypersensitivity.

C.   Type 1 diabetes is characterized by the inability of insulin-producing beta cells to fulfill their role. Usually, this happens because the immune system is attacking and destroying these cells. In other cases, a genetic problem is at the root of the problem.

D.   When supplemented shortly after birth, vitamin D dramatically reduces the chances of Type 1 diabetes developing.

E.   In type 2 diabetes several factors come into play, with beta cells ending up being damaged by an increased in blood glucose. On the one hand, regular cells become insensitive to insulin, thus requiring beta cells to produce more and more of this hormone. On the other hand, beta cells keep running out of insulin, striving to keep up with the demand for more of this hormone. At the same time, the liver regards low insulin as a sign that glucose must be low, thus releasing its blood sugar reserves. Sugar levels rise more and more to the point of damaging various areas of the body, including the beta cells themselves — perpetuating a vicious cycle of destruction.

F.   Vitamin D decreases the chances of developing type 2 diabetes. It's known that, along with vitamin K2, vitamin D increases cells' sensitivity to insulin. It's also noteworthy how the chances of developing type 2 diabetes are inversely proportional to your blood levels of vitamin D.

G. Vitamin D stimulates the immune system to attack real invaders like bacteria and viruses. Although it does not make us immune to colds and to the flu, vitamin D reduces their incidence.

H. There seems to be a link between vitamin D deficiency and fibromyalgia and chronic pain. In addition, in the case of the muscular and skeletal pain of autoimmune or inflammatory origin, vitamin D is the treatment of choice due to its rate of remission in the order of 95% obtained by the protocol of Dr. Coimbra in his clinical practice.

Chapter 12

Vitamin D and Vitamin K2 — Risks, Benefits and Secrets

Questions:

A.   What are the risks of vitamin D?

B.   What are the risks of vitamin K2?

C.   What are the benefits of vitamin D?

D.   What are the benefits of vitamin K2?

E.   What are the secrets of Vitamin D and Vitamin K2?

Answers:

A. The fundamental risks of vitamin D supplementation involve (1) an increase in blood calcium levels, (2) bone decalcification and (3) an excessive suppression of the parathyroid gland.

B. Vitamin K2 supplementation is accompanied by the theoretical risk of (1) an excessive reduction in blood calcium levels and of it (2) being converted to vitamin K1 — which could greatly harm someone under anticoagulant drug therapy.

C. Vitamin D appears to positively influence most, if not all, degenerative processes in our body.

D. Vitamin K2 is key to a good calcium metabolism. In addition, it has the extraordinary role of providing an extra safety layer regarding the use of higher doses of vitamin D.

E. One of the secrets is the synergistic relationship between vitamin D and vitamin K2. In addition, experimental protocols and several clinical studies have uncovered many other secrets regarding the ability of vitamin D to prevent, stop and even reverse some degenerative diseases.

    Other secrets involve the steps required to use the Sun, and supplementation, as a safe source of vitamin D. In the case of the Sun, these steps involve the hours you get out to get the sunlight and the care you must take to not take more sun than your skin can handle. In the case of supplementation, much care must be taken in avoiding calcium-rich food, maintaining a daily intake of 2.5 liters of fluids and keeping in mind the need for physical exercise and cofactor supplementation.

Did you know?

This book was translated and published independently. That means there is no publisher behind. This has its advantages, but one fundamental disadvantage is that there is no national marketing campaign promoting this book.

How can you help?

If you enjoyed this exploration of the secrets of vitamin D and believe in the value of the information provided, what do you think about leaving a review on Amazon? Your words will help others understand the benefits they can reap from the information contained in this book.

On the other hand, if there's any information that you don't agree with or if you need additional information, feel free to contact me at:

- tiagohenriques@vitamindanswers.com

Also, if you know about a case study or published clinical trial or another relevant piece of information you'd like to share with me, please do so.

Finally, any tips on how to improve the quality of this translation would be greatly appreciated so feel free to send me your valuable insights.

Contact me using the above email address and I'd be more than happy to read your kind words.

To conclude, I do have a **Portuguese YouTube channel**, https://www.youtube.com/c/CienciaDesenhada, where you can find instructional videos in a whiteboard animation style.

Also, I've published more research and educational material on Udemy and Amazon. However, these are currently available exclusively in Portuguese.

I have plans to eventually translate my works into English and other languages. It'll all be possible thanks to people like you. So, let me show my appreciation for the time you took to analyze this work.

I hope this valuable research can make a real difference in your health and quality of life.

Let me know how it goes for you,

Tiago Henriques

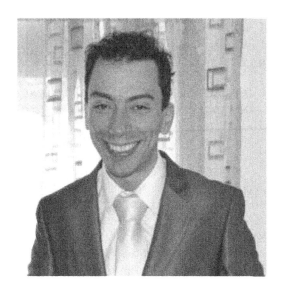

BIBLIOGRAPHIC REFERENCES

How to read the abstracts of any of the referenced studies faster: Instead of typing the full link in your browser, type only the number at the end of the link in google. The referenced study should appear as the first result.

As an example, suppose you'd like to further research reference 59:

59. Blumenthal JA, Babyak MA, Moore KA, et al. Effects of exercise training on older patients with major depression. *Arch Intern Med.* 1999;159(19):2349-56.
https://www.ncbi.nlm.nih.gov/pubmed/10547175

In this case, you would google "10547175."

As a final note, sometimes you'll find "PMC" before the number. In this case please include "PMC" in your search along with the number.

If by some reason, this method doesn't yield the results you expected just add "pubmed" to your google search.

1. Coelho MP. Chegar novo a velho, medicina do futuro. 2016. Page 134

2. Video: https://www.youtube.com/watch?v=7OzP77HtR0Q at 2 minutes and 40 seconds.

3. Chowdhury R, Kunutsor S, Vitezova A, et al. Vitamin D and risk of cause specific death: systematic review and meta-analysis of observational cohort and randomised intervention studies.
The BMJ. 2014;348:g1903. doi:10.1136/bmj.g1903.
https://www.ncbi.nlm.nih.gov/pmc/articles/PMC3972416/

4. Image: https://www.ncbi.nlm.nih.gov/pmc/articles/PMC3897595/figure/F8/

5. Image: https://www.ncbi.nlm.nih.gov/pmc/articles/PMC3897595/figure/F9/

6. Finamor DC, Sinigaglia-coimbra R, Neves LC, et al. A pilot study assessing the effect of prolonged administration of high daily doses of vitamin D on the clinical course of vitiligo and psoriasis. Dermatoendocrinol. 2013;5(1):222-34.
https://www.ncbi.nlm.nih.gov/pubmed/24494059

7. Pilz S, Dobnig H, Fischer JE, et al. Low vitamin d levels predict stroke in patients referred to coronary angiography. Stroke. 2008;39(9):2611-3. https://www.ncbi.nlm.nih.gov/pubmed/18635847

8. Garland CF, Comstock GW, Garland FC, Helsing KJ, Shaw EK, Gorham ED. Serum 25-hydroxyvitamin D and colon cancer: eight-year prospective study. Lancet. 1989;2(8673):1176-8. https://www.ncbi.nlm.nih.gov/pubmed/2572900

9. Lowe LC, Guy M, Mansi JL, et al. Plasma 25-hydroxy vitamin D concentrations, vitamin D receptor genotype and breast cancer risk in a UK Caucasian population. Eur J Cancer. 2005;41(8):1164-9.
https://www.ncbi.nlm.nih.gov/pubmed/15911240

10. Compilation of studies demonstrating the positive effects of vitamin D on cancer: http://www1.grassrootshealth.net/breast-cancer-studies

11. Holick MF, Chen TC. Vitamin D deficiency: a worldwide problem with health consequences. Am J Clin Nutr. 2008;87(4):1080S-6S.
https://www.ncbi.nlm.nih.gov/pubmed/18400738

12. Naeem Z. Vitamin D Deficiency- An Ignored Epidemic. *International Journal of Health Sciences*. 2010;4(1):V-VI.
https://www.ncbi.nlm.nih.gov/pmc/articles/PMC3068797/

13. Norman AW. From vitamin D to hormone D: fundamentals of the vitamin D endocrine system essential for good health. Am J Clin Nutr. 2008;88(2):491S-499S. https://www.ncbi.nlm.nih.gov/pubmed/18689389.

14. Herrmann W, Obeid R. Causes and Early Diagnosis of Vitamin B12 Deficiency. *Deutsches Ärzteblatt International*. 2008;105(40):680-685.
doi:10.3238/arztebl.2008.0680.

15. Holick MF, Chen TC. Vitamin D deficiency: a worldwide problem with health consequences. Am J Clin Nutr. 2008;87(4):1080S-6S.
https://www.ncbi.nlm.nih.gov/pubmed/18400738

16. Naeem Z. Vitamin D Deficiency- An Ignored Epidemic. *International Journal of Health Sciences*. 2010;4(1):V-VI.
https://www.ncbi.nlm.nih.gov/pmc/articles/PMC3068797/

17. They even gave a name to the science of name giving: onomatology.

18. Christakos S, Ajibade DV, Dhawan P, Fechner AJ, Mady LJ. Vitamin D: Metabolism. *Endocrinology and metabolism clinics of North America*. 2010;39(2):243-253. doi:10.1016/j.ecl.2010.02.002.
https://www.ncbi.nlm.nih.gov/pmc/articles/PMC2879391/

19. Each of these four chemicals is also known by many different names. You don't need to memorize them all, and diagram 2 helps us undo any confusion.

20. Article: https://www.nationalmssociety.org/What-is-MS/MS-FAQ-s#question-Is-MS-fatal

21. Video in Portuguese: https://www.youtube.com/watch?v=7OzP77HtR0Q from 2 minutes and 40 seconds

22. Video, in Portuguese:
http://sic.sapo.pt/Programas/altadefinicao/videos/2017-03-19-Alta -definition-with-Manuel Pinto-Coelho

23. Video, in Portuguese:
http://sic.sapo.pt/Programas/altadefinicao/videos/2015-05-23-Bernardo-Pinto-Coelho-em-Alta-Definicao
24. Video, in English with Portuguese subtitles:
https://www.youtube.com/watch?v=Hh8k32VsxLA
25. Video, in Portuguese: https://www.youtube.com/watch?v=hOfO29rL-gl
26. Article:
http://www.auburn.edu/academic/forestry_wildlife/fire/combustion.htm
27. Article: https://www.wired.com/2010/11/1110mars-climate-observer-report/
28. Armas LA, Hollis BW, Heaney RP. Vitamin D2 is much less effective than vitamin D3 in humans. J Clin Endocrinol Metab. 2004; 89 (11): 5387-91.
https://www.ncbi.nlm.nih.gov/pubmed/15531486
29. Article: https://ods.od.nih.gov/factsheets/VitaminD-HealthProfessional/
30. Tripković L, Lambert M, K Hart et al. Comparison of vitamin D2 and vitamin D3 supplementation in raising serum 25-hydroxyvitamin D status: a systematic review and meta-analysis. *The American Journal of Clinical Nutrition.* 2012; 95 (6): 1357-1364. doi: 10.3945 / ajcn.111.031070.
https://www.ncbi.nlm.nih.gov/pmc/articles/PMC3349454/
31. Lipkie TE, Ferruzzi MG, Weaver CM. Low bioaccessibility of vitamin D2 from yeast-fortified bread compared to crystalline D2 bread and D3 from fluid milks. Food Funct. 2016;7(11):4589-4596.
https://www.ncbi.nlm.nih.gov/pubmed/27734047
32. Keegan R-H, Lu Z, Bogusz JM, Williams JE, Holick MF. Vitamin D photobiology of mushrooms and its bioavailability in humans. *Dermato-Endocrinology.* 2013; 5 (1): 165-176. doi: 10.4161 / derm.23321.
https://www.ncbi.nlm.nih.gov/pmc/articles/PMC3897585/
33. Article:
https://dietarysupplementdatabase.usda.nih.gov/ingredient_calculator/equation.php
34. Domene AC. Multiple Sclerosis and (lots of) Vitamin D: My eight-year Treatment with The Coimbra Protocol for Autoimmune Diseases. Amazon Digital Services LLC. 2016. Page 16.
35. Goldenberg MM. Multiple Sclerosis Review. *Pharmacy and Therapeutics.* 2012; 37 (3): 175-184.
https://www.ncbi.nlm.nih.gov/pmc/articles/PMC3351877/
36. Sieper J, Braun J, M Rudwaleit Boonen A Zink A. ankylosing spondylitis: an overview. *Annals of the Rheumatic Diseases.* 2002; 61 (Suppl 3): iii18-III8. doi: 10.1136 / ard.61.suppl_3.iii8.
https://www.ncbi.nlm.nih.gov/pmc/articles/PMC1766729/
37. Hathcock JN, Shao A, Vieth R, Heaney R. Risk assessment for vitamin D. Am J Clin Nutr. 2007;85(1):6-18. https://www.ncbi.nlm.nih.gov/pubmed/17209171
38. Article: https://www.vitamindcouncil.org/about-vitamin-d/am-i-getting-too-much-vitamin-d/

39. Vieth R. Vitamin D supplementation, 25-hydroxyvitamin D concentrations, and safety. Am J Clin Nutr. 1999;69(5):842-56. https://www.ncbi.nlm.nih.gov/pubmed/10232622

40. Article: https://www.vitamindcouncil.org/about-vitamin-d/how-do-i-get-the-vitamin-d-my-body-needs/

41. Matsuoka LY, Ide L, Wortsman J, Maclaughlin JA, Holick MF. Sunscreens suppress cutaneous vitamin D3 synthesis. J Clin Endocrinol Metab. 1987;64(6):1165-8. https://www.ncbi.nlm.nih.gov/pubmed/3033008

42. Holick M. "Photobiology of Vitamin D" Vitamin D: Second Edition, 2005.

43. Article: https://www.vitamindcouncil.org/about-vitamin-d/how-do-i-get-the-vitamin-d-my-body-needs/

44. Detailed information on the amounts of vitamin D3 and D2 present in various foods is available in Appendix A.

45. Article: http://www.thisisms.com/forum/coimbra-high-dose-vitamin-d-protocol-f57/topic27182.html

46. Article: https://www.livestrong.com/article/537905-can-drinking-too-much-water-cause-low-potassium/

47. Balcı AK, Koksal O, Kose A, et al. General characteristics of patients with electrolyte imbalance admitted to emergency department. *World Journal of Emergency Medicine*. 2013;4(2):113-116. doi:10.5847/wjem.j.issn.1920-8642.2013.02.005. https://www.ncbi.nlm.nih.gov/pmc/articles/PMC4129840/

48. Weglicki W, Quamme G, Tucker K, Haigney M, Resnick L. Potassium, magnesium, and electrolyte imbalance and complications in disease management. Clin Exp Hypertens. 2005;27(1):95-112. https://www.ncbi.nlm.nih.gov/pubmed/15773233

49. Ritter CS, Armbrecht HJ, Slatopolsky E, Brown AJ. 25-Hydroxyvitamin D(3) suppresses PTH synthesis and secretion by bovine parathyroid cells. Kidney Int. 2006;70(4):654-9. https://www.ncbi.nlm.nih.gov/pubmed/16807549

50. Friedl C, Zitt E. Vitamin D prohormone in the treatment of secondary hyperparathyroidism in patients with chronic kidney disease. Int J Nephrol Renovasc Dis. 2017;10:109-122. https://www.ncbi.nlm.nih.gov/pubmed/28546765

51. Lotito A, Teramoto M, Cheung M, Becker K, Sukumar D. Serum Parathyroid Hormone Responses to Vitamin D Supplementation in Overweight/Obese Adults: A Systematic Review and Meta-Analysis of Randomized Clinical Trials. Nutrients. 2017;9(3):241. doi:10.3390/nu9030241. https://www.ncbi.nlm.nih.gov/pmc/articles/PMC5372904/

52. Abrams SA, Hawthorne KM, Chen Z. Supplementation with 1000 IU vitamin D/d leads to parathyroid hormone suppression, but not increased fractional calcium absorption, in 4-8-y-old children: a double-blind randomized controlled trial. Am J Clin Nutr. 2013;97(1):217-23. https://www.ncbi.nlm.nih.gov/pubmed/23151536

53. Tardelli VS, Lago MPPD, Silveira DXD, Fidalgo TM. Vitamin D and alcohol: A review of the current literature. Psychiatry Res. 2017;248:83-86. http://www.psy-journal.com/article/S0165-1781(16)30706-5/fulltext

54. Epstein M. Alcohol's impact on kidney function. Alcohol Health Res World. 1997;21(1):84-92.Epstein M. Alcohol's impact on kidney function. Alcohol Health Res World. 1997;21(1):84-92. https://www.ncbi.nlm.nih.gov/pubmed/15706766

55. Sampson HW. Alcohol's harmful effects on bone. Alcohol Health Res World. 1998;22(3):190-4. https://www.ncbi.nlm.nih.gov/pubmed/15706795

56. Szabo G, Mandrekar P. Focus On: Alcohol and the Liver. *Alcohol Research & Health*. 2010;33(1-2):87-96.
https://www.ncbi.nlm.nih.gov/pmc/articles/PMC3860520/

57. Zahr NM, Pfefferbaum A. Alcohol's Effects on the Brain: Neuroimaging Results in Humans and Animal Models. Alcohol Res. 2017;38(2):183-206. https://www.ncbi.nlm.nih.gov/pubmed/28988573

58. Tada A. Psychological effects of exercise on community-dwelling older adults. Clin Interv Aging. 2018;13:271-276.
https://www.ncbi.nlm.nih.gov/pubmed/29483773

59. Blumenthal JA, Babyak MA, Moore KA, et al. Effects of exercise training on older patients with major depression. Arch Intern Med. 1999;159(19):2349-56. https://www.ncbi.nlm.nih.gov/pubmed/10547175

60. Lamina S, Agbanusi E, Nwacha RC. Effects of Aerobic Exercise in the Management of Erectile Dysfunction: A Meta Analysis Study on Randomized Controlled Trials. *Ethiopian Journal of Health Sciences*. 2011;21(3):195-201. https://www.ncbi.nlm.nih.gov/pmc/articles/PMC3275865/

61. Silva AB, Sousa N, Azevedo LF, Martins C. Physical activity and exercise for erectile dysfunction: systematic review and meta-analysis. Br J Sports Med. 2017;51(19):1419-1424. https://www.ncbi.nlm.nih.gov/pubmed/27707739

62. Buchner DM, Beresford SA, Larson EB, Lacroix AZ, Wagner EH. Effects of physical activity on health status in older adults. II. Intervention studies. Annu Rev Public Health. 1992; 13:469-88.
https://www.ncbi.nlm.nih.gov/pubmed/1599599/

63. Mcmillan LB, Zengin A, Ebeling PR, Scott D. Prescribing Physical Activity for the Prevention and Treatment of Osteoporosis in Older Adults. Healthcare (Basel). 2017;5(4) https://www.ncbi.nlm.nih.gov/pubmed/29113119

64. Hinton PS, Nigh P, Thyfault J. Effectiveness of resistance training or jumping-exercise to increase bone mineral density in men with low bone mass: A 12-month randomized, clinical trial. Bone. 2015;79:203-12.
https://www.ncbi.nlm.nih.gov/pubmed/26092649

65. Zhao R, Zhao M, Zhang L. Efficiency of jumping exercise in improving bone mineral density among premenopausal women: a meta-analysis. Sports Med. 2014;44(10):1393-402. https://www.ncbi.nlm.nih.gov/pubmed/24981245

66. Paillard T. [Exercise and bone mineral density in old subjects: theorical and practical implications]. *Geriatr Psychol Neuropsychiatr Vieil*. 2014;12(3):267-73. https://www.ncbi.nlm.nih.gov/pubmed/25245313

67. Watson SL, Weeks BK, Weis LJ, Horan SA, Beck BR. Heavy resistance training is safe and improves bone, function, and stature in postmenopausal women with low to very low bone mass: novel early findings from the LIFTMOR trial. Osteoporos Int. 2015;26(12):2889-94.
https://www.ncbi.nlm.nih.gov/pubmed/26243363/

68. Brot C, Jorgensen NR, Sorensen OH. The influence of smoking on vitamin D status and calcium metabolism. Eur J Clin Nutr. 1999;53(12):920-6. https://www.ncbi.nlm.nih.gov/pubmed/10602348

69. Ren W, Gu Y, Zhu L, et al. The effect of cigarette smoking on vitamin D level and depression in male patients with acute ischemic stroke. Compr Psychiatry. 2016;65:9-14. https://www.ncbi.nlm.nih.gov/pubmed/26773985

70. Coelho MP. Chegar novo a velho, medicina do futuro. 2016. Página 134

71. Yagnik D, Serafin V, J shah A. Antimicrobial activity of apple cider vinegar against Escherichia coli, Staphylococcus aureus and Candida albicans; downregulating cytokine and microbial protein expression. Sci Rep. 2018;8(1):1732. https://www.ncbi.nlm.nih.gov/pmc/articles/PMC5788933/

72. Trill J, Simpson C, Webley F, et al. Uva-ursi extract and ibuprofen as alternative treatments of adult female urinary tract infection (ATAFUTI): study protocol for a randomised controlled trial. Trials. 2017;18(1):421. https://www.ncbi.nlm.nih.gov/pubmed/28886751

73. Hisano M, Bruschini H, Nicodemo AC, Srougi M. Cranberries and lower urinary tract infection prevention. Clinics. 2012;67(6):661-667.
doi:10.6061/clinics/2012(06)18.
https://www.ncbi.nlm.nih.gov/pmc/articles/PMC3370320/

74. Francino MP. Antibiotics and the Human Gut Microbiome: Dysbioses and Accumulation of Resistances. Frontiers in Microbiology. 2015;6:1543.
doi:10.3389/fmicb.2015.01543.
https://www.ncbi.nlm.nih.gov/pmc/articles/PMC4709861/

75. Coimbra CG, Junqueira VB. High doses of riboflavin and the elimination of dietary red meat promote the recovery of some motor functions in Parkinson's disease patients. Braz J Med Biol Res 2003; 36 (10). 1409-17. https://www.ncbi.nlm.nih.gov/pubmed/14502375

76. Anderson BB, Scattoni M, Perry GM, et al. Is the flavin-deficient red blood cell common in Maremma, Italy, an important defense against malaria in this area? American Journal of Human Genetics.1994; 55 (5): 975-980. https://www.ncbi.nlm.nih.gov/pmc/articles/PMC1918332/

77. Marashly ET, Bohlega SA. Riboflavin Has Neuroprotective Potential: Focus on Parkinson's Disease and Migraine. Front Neurol. 2017; 8: 333. https://www.ncbi.nlm.nih.gov/pmc/articles/PMC5517396/

78. Adiloğlu AK Gönülateş N, M Isler, Senol A. [The effect of kefir consumption on human immune system: to study cytokine]. Mikrobiyol Bul. 2013; 47 (2): 273-81. https://www.ncbi.nlm.nih.gov/pubmed/23621727

79. Maresz K. Calcium Proper Use: Vitamin K2 as a Promoter of Bone and Cardiovascular Health. *Integrative Medicine: A Clinician's Journal*. 2015; 14 (1): 34-39. https://www.ncbi.nlm.nih.gov/pmc/articles/PMC4566462/

80. JT Bowles. The Miraculous Results of Extremely High Doses of the Sunshine Hormone Vitamin D3 My Experiment with Huge doses of D3 from 25,000 to 50,000 to 100,000 Iu a Day Over 1 Year Period. CreateSpace; 2013.

81. Rabbit MP. Again reach old medicine of the future. 2016.

82. The Crescenti, Puiggròs F Colomé A, et al. [Antiurolithiasic effect of a mixture of Herniaria glabra plant, Agropyron repens, Equisetum arvense and Sambucus nigra (Herbensurina®) in the prevention of nephrolithiasis Experimentally induced in rats]. Arch Esp Urol. 2015; 68 (10): 739-49. https://www.ncbi.nlm.nih.gov/pubmed/26634575

83. Composition: (1) *Herniaria glabra* L. — whole plant — 1 gram per sachet. (2) *Agropyron repens* (L.) P. Beauv. — rhizome — 0.25 gram per sachet. (3) *Equisetum arvense* L. (Horsetail) — sterile stems — 0.15 grams per sachet. (4) *Sambucus nigra* L. — flower — 0.1 grams per sachet.

84. Personal communication during a consultation.

85. Bonnar J. Coagulation effects of oral contraception. Am J Obstet Gynecol. 1987; 157 (4 Pt 2): 1042-8. https://www.ncbi.nlm.nih.gov/pubmed/2960241

86. Article: https://www.sharecare.com/health/blood-basics/how-many-white-blood-cells

87. Article: https://www.healthline.com/health/how-much-blood-in-human-body

88. Article: https://www.vitamindcouncil.org/gene-expression-and-vitamin-d-whats-the-link/

89. The Nezhad-Hossein, Spira A, Holick MF. Influence of Vitamin D Status and Vitamin D3 Supplementation on Genome Wide Expression of White Blood Cells: A Randomized Double-Blind Clinical Trial. M Campbell, ed. *PLoS*ONE.2013; 8 (3): e58725. doi: 10.1371 / journal.pone.0058725.https://www.ncbi.nlm.nih.gov/pmc/articles/PMC3604145/

90. Prietl B, G Treiber, Pieber TR Amrein K. Vitamin D and Immune Function. *Nutrients.*2013; 5 (7): 2502-2521. doi: 10.3390 / nu5072502. https://www.ncbi.nlm.nih.gov/pmc/articles/PMC3738984/

91. ES Chambers, Hawrylowicz CM. The impact of vitamin D on regulatory T cells. Curr Allergy Asthma Rep 2011; 11 (1):. 29-36. https://www.ncbi.nlm.nih.gov/pubmed/21104171

92. Sigmundsdottir H, J Pan, Debes GF, et al. DCs metabolize sunlight-induced vitamin D3 to 'program' T cell attraction to the epidermal chemokine CCL27. Nat Immunol. 2007; 8 (3): 285-93. https://www.ncbi.nlm.nih.gov/pubmed/17259988

93. Pillay J, Den Braber R, Vrisekoop N, et al. In vivo labeling with 2H2 reveals the lifespan of human neutrophil 5.4 hours. Blood. 2010; 116 (4): 625-7. http://www.bloodjournal.org/content/116/4/625?ijkey=1a3c177de0b39ae4c1ec8754e0b3c71cd72451d5

94. Cvetanovich GL, Hafler DA. Regulatory T Cells in Human Autoimmune Diseases. *Current Opinion in Immunology*. 2010; 22 (6): 753-760. doi: 10.1016 / j.coi.2010.08.012. https://www.ncbi.nlm.nih.gov/pmc/articles/PMC2997859/

95. Lys K Kuzawińska O-Bałkowiec Iskra E. Tumor necrosis factor inhibitors — state of knowledge. *Archives of Medical Science:*AMS.2014; 10 (6): 1175-1185. doi: 10.5114 / aoms.2014.47827.
https://www.ncbi.nlm.nih.gov/pmc/articles/PMC4296073/

96. Article:
http://www.news.med.br/p/saude/222530/oms+divulga+as+dez+principais+causas+de+morte+no+mundo.htm

97. Sharma RK, Sharma RK, Voelker DJ, et al. Cardiac risk stratification: Role of the coronary calcium score. *Vascular Health and Risk Management*.2010; 6: 603-611. https://www.ncbi.nlm.nih.gov/pmc/articles/PMC2922321/

98. Maresz K. Calcium Proper Use: Vitamin K2 as a Promoter of Bone and Cardiovascular Health. Integrative Medicine: A Clinician's Journal. 2015; 14 (1): 34-39. https://www.ncbi.nlm.nih.gov/pmc/articles/PMC4566462/

99. Rheaume-Bleue K. Vitamin K2 and the Calcium Paradox: How a Little-Known Vitamin Could Save Your Life. Harper; 2013. page 39

100. Lhermusier T, Chap H Payrastre B. Platelet membrane phospholipid asymmetry: from the characterization of the scramblase activity to the identification of an essential protein mutated in Scott syndrome. J Thromb Haemost. 2011; 9 (10): 1883-91.
https://www.ncbi.nlm.nih.gov/pubmed/21958383

101. Haque JA, McDonald MG Kulman JD, Rettie AE. The cellular system is quantitation of vitamin K cycle activity: effects on structure-activity vitamin K warfarin metabolites by antagonism. *Blood.*2014; 123 (4): 582-589. doi: 10.1182 / blood-2013-05-505123.
https://www.ncbi.nlm.nih.gov/pmc/articles/PMC3901071/

102. Mikaelsson ME (1991) The Role of Calcium in Coagulation and Anticoagulation. In: Sibinga CTS, Das PC, Mannucci PM (eds) Coagulation and Blood Transfusion. Developments in Hematology and Immunology, vol 26. Springer, Boston, MA

103. It's noteworthy that milk and milk products such as cheese, are contraindicated in a protocol with high doses of vitamin D due to their high calcium content.

104. Tsukamoto Y, M Ichise , Kakuda H, Yamaguchi M. Intake of fermented soybean (natto) Increases circulating vitamin K2 (menaquinone-7) and gamma-carboxylated osteocalcin concentration in Normal Individuals. J Bone Miner Metab. 2000; 18 (4): 216-22. https://www.ncbi.nlm.nih.gov/pubmed/10874601

105. Article: https://pubchem.ncbi.nlm.nih.gov/compound/octane

106. Article: https://pubchem.ncbi.nlm.nih.gov/compound/ethane

107. Article: https://pubchem.ncbi.nlm.nih.gov/compound/benzene

108. Sato T, LJ Schurgers, Uenishi K. Comparison of menaquinone-4 and menaquinone-7 bioavailability in healthy women. J Nutr 2012; 11: 93. https://www.ncbi.nlm.nih.gov/pubmed/23140417

109. A fictitious vitamin.

110. This specific supplement also contains vitamin K1.

111. Conly JM, Stein K. The production of menaquinones (vitamin K2) by intestinal bacteria and their role in maintaining coagulation homeostasis. Prog Food Nutr Sci 1992; 16 (4):. 307-43. https://www.ncbi.nlm.nih.gov/pubmed/1492156

112. Bonnar J. Coagulation effects of oral contraception. Am J Obstet Gynecol. 1987; 157 (4 Pt 2): 1042-8. https://www.ncbi.nlm.nih.gov/pubmed/2960241

113. Link: https://www.ncbi.nlm.nih.gov/pubmed/?term=vitamin+D3+%2B+Depression

114. Spedding S. Vitamin D and Depression: A Systematic Review and Meta-Analysis Comparing Biological Studies With and without Flaws. *Nutrients.*2014; 6 (4): 1501-1518. doi: 10.3390 / nu6041501. https://www.ncbi.nlm.nih.gov/pmc/articles/PMC4011048/

115. Spedding S. Vitamin D and Depression: Vitamin D and Depression: A Systematic Review and Meta-Analysis Comparing Studies with and without Biological Flaws. *Nutrients.*2014; 6 (4): 1501-1518. doi: 10.3390 / nu6041501. https://www.ncbi.nlm.nih.gov/pmc/articles/PMC4011048/

116. Sartori SB N Whittle, Hetzenauer A Singewald N. Magnesium deficiency induces anxiety axis and HPA dysregulation: modulation by therapeutic drug treatment. Neuropharmacology. 2012; 62 (1): 304-12. https://www.ncbi.nlm.nih.gov/pmc/articles/PMC3198864/

117. Syed I, M Wasay, Awan S. Treating Vitamin B12 Supplementation in Major Depressive Disorder: A Randomized Controlled Trial. *The Open Neurology Journal.* 2013; 7: 44-48. doi: 10.2174 / 1874205X01307010044. https://www.ncbi.nlm.nih.gov/pmc/articles/PMC3856388/

118. Khoraminya N-Tehrani Doost M, S Jazayeri Hosseini A Djazayery A. Therapeutic effects of vitamin D therapy adjunctive to the fluoxetine in Patients with major depressive disorder. Aust NZJ Psychiatry. 2013; 47 (3): 271-5. https://www.ncbi.nlm.nih.gov/pubmed/23093054

119. Gloth FM Alam W, Hollis B. Vitamin D vs. broad spectrum phototherapy in the treatment of seasonal affective disorder. J Nutr Health Aging. 1999; 3 (1): 5-7. https://www.ncbi.nlm.nih.gov/pubmed/10888476

120. Gancheva SM, Zhelyazkova-Savova MD. Vitamin K2 Improves Anxiety and Depression but not Cognition in Rats with Metabolic Syndrome: The Role of Blood Glucose ?. Folia Med (Plovdiv). 2016; 58 (4): 264-272. https://www.ncbi.nlm.nih.gov/pubmed/28068285

121. An analogy popularized by autistic author Temple Grandin

122. Jia F, B Wang, Shan L, Xu Z, WG Staal, L. Du Core Symptoms of Vitamin D autism improved after supplementation. Pediatrics. 2015; 135 (1): e196-8. https://www.ncbi.nlm.nih.gov/pubmed/25511123

123. Cannell JJ. Vitamin D and autism, what's new ?. Rev Endocr Metab Disord. 2017; 18 (2): 183-193. https://www.ncbi.nlm.nih.gov/pubmed/28217829

124. Cannell JJ, Grant WB. What is the role of Vitamin D in autism ?. Dermatoendocrinol. 2013; 5 (1): 199-204. https://www.ncbi.nlm.nih.gov/pubmed/24494055

125. Article: https://www.ncbi.nlm.nih.gov/pubmedhealth/PMHT0024869/

126. Stubbs G, Henley K, Green J. Autism: Will vitamin D supplementation during pregnancy and early childhood reduces the recurrence rate of autism in newborn siblings ?. Med Hypotheses. 2016; 88: 74-8. https://www.ncbi.nlm.nih.gov/pubmed/26880644

127. Saad K, Abdel-Rahman AA, Elserogy YM, et al. Vitamin D status in autism spectrum disorders and the efficacy of vitamin D supplementation in autistic children. Nutr Neurosci. 2016: 19 (8): 346-351. https://www.ncbi.nlm.nih.gov/pubmed/25876214

128. Link: www.vitamindcouncil.org

129. Cannell JJ. Autism and vitamin D. Med Hypotheses. 2008; 70 (4): 750-9. https://www.ncbi.nlm.nih.gov/pubmed/17920208

130. Cannell JJ. Autism, will vitamin D treat core symptoms ?. Med Hypotheses. 2013; 81 (2): 195-8. https://www.ncbi.nlm.nih.gov/pubmed/23725905

131. Spedding S. Vitamin D and Depression: A Systematic Review and Meta-Analysis Comparing Studies with and without Biological Flaws. *Nutrients*. 2014; 6 (4): 1501-1518. doi: 10.3390 / nu6041501. https://www.ncbi.nlm.nih.gov/pmc/articles/PMC4011048/

132. Cannell JJ. Autism and vitamin D. Med Hypotheses. 2008; 70 (4): 750-9. https://www.ncbi.nlm.nih.gov/pubmed/17920208

133. Article: https://www.medscape.com/viewarticle/551998

134. Fouad YA, Aanei C. Revisiting the hallmarks of cancer. *American Journal of Cancer Research*. 2017; 7 (5): 1016-1036. https://www.ncbi.nlm.nih.gov/pmc/articles/PMC5446472/

135. Chakraborti CK. Vitamin D as a promising anticancer agent. *Indian Journal of Pharmacology*. 2011; 43 (2): 113-120. doi: 10.4103 / 0253-7613.77335. https://www.ncbi.nlm.nih.gov/pmc/articles/PMC3081446/

136. LC Lowe, Guy F, Mansi JL, et al. Plasma 25-hydroxy Vitamin D Concentrations, vitamin D receptor genotype and breast cancer risk in the UK Caucasian population. Eur J Cancer. 2005; 41 (8): 1164-9. https://www.ncbi.nlm.nih.gov/pubmed/15911240

137. Garland CF, Comstock GW, Garland FC, Helsing KJ, EK Shaw, Gorham ED. Serum 25-hydroxyvitamin D and colon cancer: eight-year prospective study. Lancet. 1989; 2 (8673): 1176-8. https://www.ncbi.nlm.nih.gov/pubmed/2572900/

138. Der T, BA Bailey, D Youssef, Manning T, Grant WB, Peiris AN. Vitamin D and prostate cancer survival in veterans. Mil Med 2014; 179 (1):. 81-4. https://www.ncbi.nlm.nih.gov/pubmed/24402990

139. Norton R O'Connell MA. Vitamin D: potential in the prevention and treatment of lung cancer. Anticancer Res 2012; 32 (1):. 211-21. https://www.ncbi.nlm.nih.gov/pubmed/22213310

140. Kiely M Hodgins SJ Merrigan BA, S Tormey, PA Kiely, O'Connor. Real-time cell analysis of the inhibitory effect of vitamin K2 on adhesion and proliferation of breast cancer cells. Nutr Res 2015; 35 (8):. 736-43. https://www.ncbi.nlm.nih.gov/pubmed/26082424

141. Shibayama Imazu-T, T Aiuchi, Nakaya K. Vitamin K2-mediated apoptosis in cancer cells: role of mitochondrial transmembrane potential. Vitam Horm. 2008; 78: 211-26. https://www.ncbi.nlm.nih.gov/pubmed/18374196

142. F Duan, Yu Y, Guan R, Z Xu, Liang H, Hong L. Vitamin K2 Induces Apoptosis-Related Mitochondria in Human Bladder Cancer Cells via ROS and JNK / p38 MAPK Pathways Signal. YH Hsieh, ed. *PLoS*ONE.2016; 11 (8): e0161886. doi: 10.1371 / journal.pone.0161886. https://www.ncbi.nlm.nih.gov/pmc/articles/PMC5003392/

143. The Samykutty, Shetty AV Dakshinamoorthy G, et al. Vitamin K2, the naturally occurring Menaquinone, Exerts Both Therapeutic Effects on Hormone-Dependent and Independent Prostate Cancer Hormone-Cells. *Evidence-Based Complementary and Alternative Medicine:*eCAM.2013; 2013: 287358. doi: 10.1155 / 2013/287358. https://www.ncbi.nlm.nih.gov/pmc/articles/PMC3767046/

144. Tokita H, Tsuchida A Miyazawa K, et al. Vitamin K2-induced antitumor effects via cell-cycle arrest and apoptosis in gastric cancer cell lines. Int J Mol Med 2006; 17 (2):. 235-43. https://www.ncbi.nlm.nih.gov/pubmed/16391821

145. Matsumoto K, J Okano, T Nagahara, Y. Murawaki Apoptosis of liver cancer cells by vitamin K2 and enhancement by MEK inhibition. Int J Oncol. 2006; 29 (6): 1501-8. https://www.ncbi.nlm.nih.gov/pubmed/17088989

146. Xia JB, Wang CZ, Ma JX, An XJ. [Immunoregulatory role of 1, 25-dihydroxyvitamin D(3)-treated dendritic cells in allergic airway inflammation]. Zhonghua Yi Xue Za Zhi. 2009;89(8):514-8. https://www.ncbi.nlm.nih.gov/pubmed/19567068

147. Sandhu MS, Casale TB. The role of vitamin D in asthma. Ann Allergy Asthma Immunol. 2010;105(3):191-9. https://www.ncbi.nlm.nih.gov/pubmed/20800785

148. Yadav M, Mittal K. Effect of vitamin D supplementation on moderate to severe bronchial asthma. Indian J Pediatr. 2014;81(7):650-4. https://www.ncbi.nlm.nih.gov/pubmed/24193954/

149. Ali NS, Nanji K. A Review on the Role of Vitamin D in Asthma. Muacevic A, Adler JR, eds. *Cureus.* 2017;9(5):e1288. doi:10.7759/cureus.1288. https://www.ncbi.nlm.nih.gov/pmc/articles/PMC5491340/

150. Kimur I, Tanizaki Y, Sato S, Saito K, Takahashi K. Menaquinone (vitamin K2) therapy for bronchial asthma. II. Clinical effect of menaquinone on bronchial asthma. Acta Med Okayama. 1975;29(2):127-35. https://www.ncbi.nlm.nih.gov/pubmed/51576

151. Abou-Hamdan M, Gharib B, Bajenoff M, Julia V, de Reggi M. Pantethine Down-Regulates Leukocyte Recruitment and Inflammatory Parameters in a Mouse Model of Allergic Airway Inflammation. *Medical Science Monitor Basic Research*. 2017;23:368-372. doi:10.12659/MSMBR.904077. https://www.ncbi.nlm.nih.gov/pmc/articles/PMC5717997/

152. Article: https://labtestsonline.org.br/tests/glicose

153. Hyppönen E, Läärä E, Reunanen A, Järvelin MR, Virtanen SM. Intake of vitamin D and risk of type 1 diabetes: a birth-cohort study. Lancet. 2001;358(9292):1500-3. https://www.ncbi.nlm.nih.gov/pubmed/11705562

154. Vitamin D and Diabetes. Teresa Martin, R. Keith Campbell. Diabetes Spectrum May 2011, 24 (2) 113-118; DOI: 10.2337/diaspect.24.2.113 http://spectrum.diabetesjournals.org/content/24/2/113

155. Zeitz U, Weber K, Soegiarto DW, Wolf E, Balling R, Erben RG. Impaired insulin secretory capacity in mice lacking a functional vitamin D receptor. FASEB J. 2003;17(3):509-11. https://www.ncbi.nlm.nih.gov/pubmed/12551842

156. Iwamoto J, Sato Y, Takeda T, Matsumoto H. Bone quality and vitamin K2 in type 2 diabetes: review of preclinical and clinical studies. Nutr Rev. 2011;69(3):162-7. https://www.ncbi.nlm.nih.gov/pubmed/21348880

157. Li Y, Chen JP, Duan L, Li S. Effect of vitamin K2 on type 2 diabetes mellitus: A review. Diabetes Res Clin Pract. 2018;136:39-51. https://www.ncbi.nlm.nih.gov/pubmed/29196151

158. Manna P, Kalita J. Beneficial role of vitamin K supplementation on insulin sensitivity, glucose metabolism, and the reduced risk of type 2 diabetes: A review. Nutrition. 2016;32(7-8):732-9. https://www.ncbi.nlm.nih.gov/pubmed/27133809

159. Wei J, Karsenty G. An overview of the metabolic functions of osteocalcin. Rev Endocr Metab Disord. 2015;16(2):93-8. https://www.ncbi.nlm.nih.gov/pubmed/25577163

160. Choi HJ, Yu J, Choi H, et al. Vitamin K2 supplementation improves insulin sensitivity via osteocalcin metabolism: a placebo-controlled trial. Diabetes Care. 2011;34(9):e147.http://care.diabetesjournals.org/content/34/9/e147

161. Article: https://news.harvard.edu/gazette/story/2017/02/study-confirms-vitamin-d-protects-against-cold-and-flu/

162. Sabetta JR, Depetrillo P, Cipriani RJ, Smardin J, Burns LA, Landry ML. Serum 25-hydroxyvitamin d and the incidence of acute viral respiratory tract infections in healthy adults. PLoS ONE. 2010;5(6):e11088. https://www.ncbi.nlm.nih.gov/pubmed/20559424

163. Clauw DJ. Fibromyalgia: a clinical review. JAMA. 2014;311(15):1547-55. https://www.ncbi.nlm.nih.gov/pubmed/24737367

164. Bellato E, Marini E, Castoldi F, et al. Fibromyalgia Syndrome: Etiology, Pathogenesis, Diagnosis, and Treatment. *Pain Research and Treatment*. 2012;2012:426130. doi:10.1155/2012/426130. https://www.ncbi.nlm.nih.gov/pmc/articles/PMC3503476/

165. Article: https://www.mayoclinic.org/diseases-conditions/fibromyalgia/symptoms-causes/syc-20354780

166. Tague SE, Clarke GL, Winter MK, McCarson KE, Wright DE, Smith PG. Vitamin D Deficiency Promotes Skeletal Muscle Hypersensitivity and Sensory Hyperinnervation. The Journal of Neuroscience. 2011;31(39):13728-13738. doi:10.1523/JNEUROSCI.3637-11.2011.
https://www.ncbi.nlm.nih.gov/pmc/articles/PMC3319727/
167. Bhatty SA, Shaikh NA, Irfan M, et al. Vitamin D deficiency in fibromyalgia. J Pak Med Assoc. 2010;60(11):949-51.
https://www.ncbi.nlm.nih.gov/pubmed/21375201
168. Dogru A, Balkarli A, Cobankara V, Tunc SE, Sahin M. Effects of Vitamin D Therapy on Quality of Life in Patients with Fibromyalgia. The Eurasian Journal of Medicine. 2017;49(2):113-117. doi:10.5152/eurasianjmed.2017.16283.
https://www.ncbi.nlm.nih.gov/pmc/articles/PMC5469836/
169. Shipton EA, Shipton EE. Vitamin D and Pain: Vitamin D and Its Role in the Aetiology and Maintenance of Chronic Pain States and Associated Comorbidities. Pain Res Treat. 2015;2015:904967.
https://www.hindawi.com/journals/prt/2015/904967/
170. Staines DR. Is fibromyalgia an autoimmune disorder of endogenous vasoactive neuropeptides?. Med Hypotheses. 2004;62(5):665-9.
https://www.ncbi.nlm.nih.gov/pubmed/15082086
171. Mcbeth J, Jones K. Epidemiology of chronic musculoskeletal pain. Best Pract Res Clin Rheumatol. 2007;21(3):403-25.
https://www.ncbi.nlm.nih.gov/pubmed/17602991/
172. Alvarez DJ, Rockwell PG. Trigger points: diagnosis and management. Am Fam Physician. 2002;65(4):653-60. https://www.ncbi.nlm.nih.gov/pubmed/11871683
173. Knutsen KV, Brekke M, Gjelstad S, Lagerløv P. Vitamin D status in patients with musculoskeletal pain, fatigue and headache: a cross-sectional descriptive study in a multi-ethnic general practice in Norway. Scand J Prim Health Care. 2010;28(3):166-71. https://www.ncbi.nlm.nih.gov/pubmed/20642395
174. Wang H, Chen W, Li D, et al. Vitamin D and Chronic Diseases. Aging and Disease. 2017;8(3):346-353. doi:10.14336/AD.2016.1021.
https://www.ncbi.nlm.nih.gov/pmc/articles/PMC5440113/
175. Article: https://www.endocrinology.org/press/press-releases/vitamin-d-may-be-simple-treatment-to-enhance-burn-healing/
176. Link: https://www.usda.gov/
177. Tsukamoto Y, Ichise H, Kakuda H, Yamaguchi M. Intake of fermented soybean (natto) increases circulating vitamin K2 (menaquinone-7) and gamma-carboxylated osteocalcin concentration in normal individuals. J Bone Miner Metab. 2000; 18 (4): 216-22. https://www.ncbi.nlm.nih.gov/pubmed/10874601
178. Link: https://www.usda.gov/
179. Link:
http://www2.insa.pt/sites/INSA/Portugues/AreasCientificas/AlimentNutricao/Aplicacoes Online/TabelaAlimentos/Paginas/TabelaAlimentos.aspx
180. Link: http://portfir.insa.pt/

181. Article: https://www.mayomedicallaboratories.com/test-catalog/Clinical+and+Interpretive/9154

182. TheOsimani, Berger, Friedman J, Katz BS-Porat, Abarbanel JM. Neuropsychology of vitamin B12 deficiency in elderly dementia patients and control subjects. J Geriatr Psychiatry Neurol. 2005; 18 (1): 33-8. https://www.ncbi.nlm.nih.gov/pubmed/15681626

183. Oudshoorn C, Mattace-raso FU, Van der velde N, Colin EM, Van der cammen TJ. Higher serum vitamin D3 levels are associated with better cognitive performance in patients with Alzheimer's disease. Dement Geriatr Cogn Disord. 2008; 25 (6): 539-43. https://www.ncbi.nlm.nih.gov/pubmed/18503256

184. Article: http://newsroom.ucla.edu/releases/ucla-study-finds-vitamin-d-may-94903

185. Lin L, Huang QX, Yang SS, Chu J, Wang JZ, Tian Q. Melatonin in Alzheimer's Disease. International Journal of Molecular Sciences. 2013; 14 (7): 14575-14593. doi: 10.3390/ijms140714575. https://www.ncbi.nlm.nih.gov/pmc/articles/PMC3742260/

186. Watanabe F, Yabuta Y, Bito T, Teng F. Vitamin B12-Containing Plant Food Sources for Vegetarians. Nutrients. 2014; 6 (5): 1861-1873. doi: 10.3390/nu6051861. https://www.ncbi.nlm.nih.gov/pmc/articles/PMC4042564/

187. Kumudha A, Selvakumar S, Dilshad P, Vaidyanathan G, Thakur MS, Sarada R. Methylcobalamin - the form of vitamin B12 identified and characterized in Chlorella vulgaris. Food Chem. 2015; 170: 316-20. https://www.ncbi.nlm.nih.gov/pubmed/25306351

188. Article: https://www.mayomedicallaboratories.com/test-catalog/Clinical+and+Interpretive/8822

189. Article: https://emedicine.medscape.com/article/2088672-overview

190. Article: http://www.labtestsonline-pt.org/tests/VitaminD.html?tab=2

191. Article: https://www.linkedin.com/pulse/125oh2d-calcitriol-reference-ranges-meg-mangin-rn/

192. Brot C, Jorgensen NR, Sorensen OH. The influence of smoking on vitamin D status and calcium metabolism. Eur J Clin Nutr. 1999; 53 (12): 920-6. https://www.ncbi.nlm.nih.gov/pubmed/10602348

193. Bell NH, Shaw S, Turner RT. Evidence that 1,25-dihydroxyvitamin D3 inhibits the hepatic production of 25-hydroxyvitamin D in man. J Clin Invest. 1984; 74 (4): 1540-4. https://www.ncbi.nlm.nih.gov/pubmed/6332830

194. Article: https://mpkb.org/home/tests/125d

195. Article: https://www.mayomedicallaboratories.com/test-catalog/Clinical+and+Interpretive/8822

196. Article: https://www.nhlbi.nih.gov/health-topics/sarcoidosis

197. Article: https://www.msdmanuals.com/en/professional/immunology-disturbances-all-country/imunodeficiencies/doen%C3%A7a-granulomatosa-cr%C3% B4nica-dgc

198. Chambourlier P, Weiller PJ, Gabriel B, Mongin M. [Vitamin D hypersensitivity is a reality in sarcoidosis]. Nouv Presse Med. 1979; 8 (10): 784. https://www.ncbi.nlm.nih.gov/pubmed/461127

199. Article: http://www.sbpc.org.br/noticias-e-comunicacao/novos-intervalos-de-referencia-de-vitamina-d/

200. Article: https://www.mayomedicallaboratories.com/test-catalog/Clinical+and+Interpretive/83670

201. Article: https://www.vitamindcouncil.org/for-health-professionals-position-statement-on-supplementation-blood-levels-and-sun-exposure/

202. Article: https://emedicine.medscape.com/article/2089334-overview

203. Article: https://emedicine.medscape.com/article/2087447-overview

204. Article: https://labtestsonline.org.br/tests/calcio

205. Article: https://labtestsonline.org.br/tests/calcio

206. Article: https://medlineplus.gov/ency/article/003474.htm

207. Article: https://www.mundovestibular.com.br/articles/964/1/NITROGENIO-UREICO-SANGUINEO-BUN/Paacutegina1.html

208. Article: https://emedicine.medscape.com/article/2054342-overview

209. Article: https://emedicine.medscape.com/article/2054430-overview

210. Article: http://www.saudedireta.com.br/docsupload/1335440721Fasc2_laboratorial_parte_002.pdf

211. Article: http://www.alvaro.com.br/laboratorio/menu-exames/FERRI

212. Ren Y, Walczyk T. Quantification of ferritin bound iron in human serum using species-specific isotope dilution mass spectrometry. Metallomics. 2014;6(9):1709-17. https://www.ncbi.nlm.nih.gov/pubmed/25008269

213. Article: https://www.mayomedicallaboratories.com/test-catalog/Clinical+and+Interpretive/8638

214. Vincent JB. Chromium: celebrating 50 years as an essential element?. Dalton Trans. 2010;39(16):3787-94. https://www.ncbi.nlm.nih.gov/pubmed/20372701

215. Vincent JB. Chromium: is it essential, pharmacologically relevant, or toxic?. Met Ions Life Sci. 2013;13:171-98.
https://www.ncbi.nlm.nih.gov/pubmed/24470092

216. Schachter S, Nelson RW, Kirk CA. Oral chromium picolinate and control of glycemia in insulin-treated diabetic dogs. J Vet Intern Med. 2001;15(4):379-84. https://www.ncbi.nlm.nih.gov/pubmed/11467597

217. Vincent JB. New Evidence against Chromium as an Essential Trace Element. J Nutr. 2017;147(12):2212-2219.
https://www.ncbi.nlm.nih.gov/pubmed/29021369

218. Ashoush S, Abou-gamrah A, Bayoumy H, Othman N. Chromium picolinate reduces insulin resistance in polycystic ovary syndrome: Randomized controlled trial. J Obstet Gynaecol Res. 2016;42(3):279-85.
https://www.ncbi.nlm.nih.gov/pubmed/26663540

219. Drake TC, Rudser KD, Seaquist ER, Saeed A. Chromium infusion in hospitalized patients with severe insulin resistance: a retrospective analysis.

Endocr Pract. 2012;18(3):394-8.
https://www.ncbi.nlm.nih.gov/pubmed/22297054

220. Broadhurst CL, Domenico P. Clinical studies on chromium picolinate supplementation in diabetes mellitus—a review. Diabetes Technol Ther. 2006;8(6):677-87. https://www.ncbi.nlm.nih.gov/pubmed/17109600

221. Cerulli J, Grabe DW, Gauthier I, Malone M, Mcgoldrick MD. Chromium picolinate toxicity. Ann Pharmacother. 1998;32(4):428-31. https://www.ncbi.nlm.nih.gov/pubmed/9562138

222. Article: https://www.mayomedicallaboratories.com/test-catalog/Clinical+and+Interpretive/8408

223. Article: https://medlineplus.gov/ency/article/003506.htm

224. Article: https://www.mayomedicallaboratories.com/test-catalog/Clinical+and+Interpretive/60475

225. Article: https://www.mayomedicallaboratories.com/test-catalog/Clinical+and+Interpretive/9265

226. Khan AP, Rajendiran TM, Ateeq B, et al. The Role of Sarcosine Metabolism in Prostate Cancer Progression. Neoplasia (New York, NY). 2013;15(5):491-501. https://www.ncbi.nlm.nih.gov/pubmed/23633921

227. Burtis CA, Bruns DE. Tietz Fundamentos de Química Clínica e Diagnóstico Molecular. Elsevier; 2016.

228. Article: https://www.mayoclinic.org/tests-procedures/liver-function-tests/about/pac-20394595

229. Article: https://emedicine.medscape.com/article/2087247-overview

230. Article: https://www.mayoclinic.org/tests-procedures/liver-function-tests/about/pac-20394595

231. Ramati E, Israel A, Tal kessler, et al. [Low ALT activity amongst patients hospitalized in internal medicine wards is a widespread phenomenon associated with low vitamin B6 levels in their blood]. Harefuah. 2015;154(2):89-93, 137. https://www.ncbi.nlm.nih.gov/pubmed/25856859

232. Article: https://emedicine.medscape.com/article/2074091-overview

233. Article: https://minutosaudavel.com.br/o-que-e-tsh-alto-e-baixo-valores-de-referencia-e-exame-de-tsh/#preparacao

234. Maxon HR, Apple DJ, Goldsmith RE. Hypercalcemia in thyrotoxicosis. Surg Gynecol Obstet. 1978;147(5):694-6. https://www.ncbi.nlm.nih.gov/pubmed/715646

235. Osman malik Y, Raza SM, Arunselvan S. Coexisting tertiary hyperparathyroidism and severe hypothyroidism in an end-stage renal disease patient on hemodialysis. Nephrourol Mon. 2015;7(2):e27191. https://www.ncbi.nlm.nih.gov/pubmed/25883915

236. Anastasilakis AD, Polyzos SA, Karathanasi E, Efstathiadou Z. Coincidence of severe primary hyperparathyroidism and primary hypothyroidism in a postmenopausal woman with low bone mass—initial conservative management. J Musculoskelet Neuronal Interact. 2011;11(1):77-80.

https://www.ncbi.nlm.nih.gov/pubmed/21364276. The complete study can be accessed here: http://www.ismni.org/jmni/pdf/43/08ANASTASILAKIS_CQ.pdf

237. Article: https://www.mayomedicallaboratories.com/test-catalog/Clinical+and+Interpretive/82985

238. Article: https://www.sciencedirect.com/topics/medicine-and-dentistry/osteoblast

239. Article: https://www.mayomedicallaboratories.com/test-catalog/Clinical+and+Interpretive/61695

240. Udhayakumar S, Shankar KG, Sowndarya S, Rose C. Novel fibrous collagen-based cream accelerates fibroblast growth for wound healing applications: in vitro and in vivo evaluation. Biomater Sci. 2017: 5 (9): 1868-1883. https://www.ncbi.nlm.nih.gov/pubmed/28676877

241. Article: http://www.scielo.br/scielo.php?script=sci_arttext&pid=S0104-42301997000400016

242. Dean-Colomb W, Hess KR, Young E, et al. Elevated serum P1NP predicts development of bone metastasis and survival in early-stage breast cancer. Breast cancer research and treatment. 2013; 137 (2): 10,1007 / s10549-012-2374-0. doi: 10.1007 / s10549-012-2374-0. https://www.ncbi.nlm.nih.gov/pmc/articles/PMC3867793/

243. Article: http://www.hermespardini.com.br/scripts/mgwms32.dll?MGWLPN=HPHOSTBS&App=HELPE&EXAME=S%7C%7CCTX

244. If you want a simple mnemonic to never confuse the two, imagine that the osteoblast blows (blasts) particles of bone tissue to form bone, just like an ink gun. At the same time imagine the osteoclast carrying an ax and "clashing" away bone tissue. Remember: osteo**BLASTS** build bone and osteo**CLAST**s strip bone away.

245. Badel T, Pavicin IS, Carek AJ, Rosin-Grget K, Grbesa D. Pathophysiology of osteonecrosis of the jaw in patients treated with bisphosphonate. Coll Antropol. 2013; 37 (2): 645-51. https://www.ncbi.nlm.nih.gov/pubmed/23941019

246. A review of the literature on osteonecrosis of patients with osteoporosis treated with oral bisphosphonates: prevalence, risk factors, and clinical characteristics. Clin Ther. 2007; 29 (8): 1548-58. https://www.ncbi.nlm.nih.gov/pubmed/17919538

247. Article: https://emedicine.medscape.com/article/2093999-overview#a2

248. Article: https://emedicine.medscape.com/article/2087447-overview

249. Domene, AC. Multiple Sclerosis and (lots of) Vitamin D: My Eight-Year Treatment with The Coimbra Protocol for Autoimmune Diseases. Amazon Digital Services LLC. 2016. Page 17.

250. Composition: (1) *Herniaria glabra L.* — whole plant — 1 gram per sachet. (2) *Agropyron repens (L.) P. Beauv.* — rhizome — 0.25 gram per sachet. (3) *Equisetum arvense L. (*Horsetail*)* — sterile stems — 0.15 grams per sachet. (4) *Sambucus nigra L.* — flower — 0.1 grams per sachet.

251. Article: https://www.mayomedicallaboratories.com/test-catalog/Clinical+and+Interpretive/8526

252. Article: https://www.mayomedicallaboratories.com/test-catalog/Clinical+and+Interpretive/81692

253. Article: https://www.mayomedicallaboratories.com/test-catalog/Clinical+and+Interpretive/81390

254. Article: https://www.mayomedicallaboratories.com/test-catalog/Clinical%20and%20Interpretive/8460

255. Article: https://www.mayomedicallaboratories.com/test-catalog/Clinical+and+Interpretive/8448

256. Article: https://www.mayomedicallaboratories.com/test-catalog/Clinical+and+Interpretive/876

257. Chang CY, Ke DS, Chen JY. Essential fatty acids and human brain. Acta Neurol Taiwan. 2009; 18 (4): 231-41. https://www.ncbi.nlm.nih.gov/pubmed/20329590

258. Mousavi nasl-khameneh A, Mirshafiey A, Naser moghadasi A, et al. Combination treatment of docosahexaenoic acid (DHA) and all-trans-retinoic acid (ATRA) inhibit IL-17 and RORγt gene expression in PBMCs of patients with relapsing-remitting multiple sclerosis. Neurol Res. 2018; 40 (1): 11-17. https://www.ncbi.nlm.nih.gov/pubmed/29155646

259. Article: https://en.wikipedia.org/wiki/MacGyver_(1985_TV_series)#%22MacGyver%22_and_%22MacGyverism%22

260. Article: https://www.mayoclinic.org/drugs-supplements/zinc-supplement-oral-route-parenteral-route/proper-use/drg -20070269

261. Prasad AS. Zinc in human health: effect of zinc on immune cells. Mol Med. 2008;14(5-6):353-7. https://www.ncbi.nlm.nih.gov/pubmed/18385818

262. Gammoh NZ, Rink L. Zinc in Infection and Inflammation. Nutrients. 2017;9(6):624. doi:10.3390/nu9060624. https://www.ncbi.nlm.nih.gov/pmc/articles/PMC5490603/

263. Haase H, Rink L. Zinc signals and immune function. Biofactors. 2014;40(1):27-40. https://www.ncbi.nlm.nih.gov/pubmed/23804522/

264. Roohani N, Hurrell R, Kelishadi R, Schulin R. Zinc and its importance for human health: An integrative review. Journal of Research in Medical Sciences : The Official Journal of Isfahan University of Medical Sciences. 2013;18(2):144-157. https://www.ncbi.nlm.nih.gov/pmc/articles/PMC3724376/

265. Barrie SA, Wright JV, Pizzorno JE, Kutter E, Barron PC. Comparative absorption of zinc picolinate, zinc citrate and zinc gluconate in humans. Agents Actions. 1987;21(1-2):223-8. https://www.ncbi.nlm.nih.gov/pubmed/3630857

266. Zeisel SH, Da costa KA. Choline: an essential nutrient for public health. Nutr Rev. 2009;67(11):615-23. https://www.ncbi.nlm.nih.gov/pubmed/19906248

267. Sanders LM, Zeisel SH. Choline: Dietary Requirements and Role in Brain Development. Nutrition today. 2007;42(4):181-186. doi:10.1097/01.NT.0000286155.55343.fa. https://www.ncbi.nlm.nih.gov/pmc/articles/PMC2518394/

268. Zeisel SH. Dietary Choline Deficiency causes DNA Strand Breaks and Alters Epigenetic Marks on DNA and Histones. Mutation Research. 2012;733(1-2):34-38. doi:10.1016/j.mrfmmm.2011.10.008.
https://www.ncbi.nlm.nih.gov/pmc/articles/PMC3319504/

269. Wu P, Jiang J, Liu Y, et al. Dietary choline modulates immune responses, and gene expressions of TOR and eIF4E-binding protein2 in immune organs of juvenile Jian carp (Cyprinus carpio var. Jian). Fish Shellfish Immunol. 2013;35(3):697-706.
https://www.ncbi.nlm.nih.gov/pubmed/23774323

270. Zeisel SH. Nutritional importance of choline for brain development. J Am Coll Nutr. 2004;23(6 Suppl):621S-626S.
https://www.ncbi.nlm.nih.gov/pubmed/15640516

271. Skripuletz T, Manzel A, Gropengießer K, et al. Pivotal role of choline metabolites in remyelination. Brain. 2015;138(Pt 2):398-413.
https://www.ncbi.nlm.nih.gov/pubmed/25524711

272. Article: https://www.pharmacistanswers.com/questions/do-you-need-to-take-magnesium-with-food

273. Oyarzúa alarcón P, Sossa K, Contreras D, Urrutia H, Nocker A. Antimicrobial properties of magnesium chloride at low pH in the presence of anionic bases. Magnes Res. 2014;27(2):57-68.
https://www.ncbi.nlm.nih.gov/pubmed/25252874

274. Jahnen-dechent W, Ketteler M. Magnesium basics. Clin Kidney J. 2012;5(Suppl 1):i3-i14.
https://www.ncbi.nlm.nih.gov/pmc/articles/PMC4455825/

275. Wanli Guo, Hussain Nazim, Zongsuo Liang, Dongfeng Yang, Magnesium deficiency in plants: An urgent problem, The Crop Journal, Volume 4, Issue 2, 2016, Pages 83-91, ISSN 2214-5141
https://www.sciencedirect.com/science/article/pii/S221451411500121X

276. Johnson S. The multifaceted and widespread pathology of magnesium deficiency. Med Hypotheses. 2001;56(2):163-70.
https://www.ncbi.nlm.nih.gov/pubmed/11425281

277. Houston M. The role of magnesium in hypertension and cardiovascular disease. J Clin Hypertens (Greenwich). 2011;13(11):843-7.
https://www.ncbi.nlm.nih.gov/pubmed/22051430

278. Stanislavov R, Nikolova V. Treatment of erectile dysfunction with pycnogenol and L-arginine. J Sex Marital Ther. 2003;29(3):207-13.
https://www.ncbi.nlm.nih.gov/pubmed/12851125

279. Pearson PJ, Evora PR, Seccombe JF, Schaff HV. Hypomagnesemia inhibits nitric oxide release from coronary endothelium: protective role of magnesium infusion after cardiac operations. Ann Thorac Surg. 1998;65(4):967-72.
https://www.ncbi.nlm.nih.gov/pubmed/9564911

280. Talib RA, Khalafalla K, Cangüven Ö. The role of vitamin D supplementation on erectile function. Turkish Journal of Urology. 2017;43(2):105-111. doi:10.5152/tud.2017.76032.
https://www.ncbi.nlm.nih.gov/pmc/articles/PMC5503426/

281. Article: http://www.lifeextension.com/Magazine/2017/10/Longevity-Benefits-of-Magnesium/Page-01

282. Abraham KJ, Chan JNY, Salvi JS, et al. Intersection of calorie restriction and magnesium in the suppression of genome-destabilizing RNA–DNA hybrids. Nucleic Acids Research. 2016;44(18):8870-8884. doi:10.1093/nar/gkw752. https://www.ncbi.nlm.nih.gov/pmc/articles/PMC5063000/

283. Mirmalek SA, Jangholi E, Jafari M, et al. Comparison of in Vitro Cytotoxicity and Apoptogenic Activity of Magnesium Chloride and Cisplatin as Conventional Chemotherapeutic Agents in the MCF-7 Cell Line. Asian Pac J Cancer Prev. 2016;17(S3):131-4. https://www.ncbi.nlm.nih.gov/pubmed/27165250

284. Coimbra CG, Junqueira VB. High doses of riboflavin and the elimination of dietary red meat promote the recovery of some motor functions in Parkinson's disease patients. Braz J Med Biol Res 2003; 36 (10). 1409-17. https://www.ncbi.nlm.nih.gov/pubmed/14502375

285. Anderson BB, Scattoni M, Perry GM, et al. Is the flavin-deficient red blood cell common in Maremma, Italy, an important defense against malaria in this area? *American Journal of Human Genetics*.1994; 55 (5): 975-980. https://www.ncbi.nlm.nih.gov/pmc/articles/PMC1918332/

286. Marashly ET, Bohlega SA. Riboflavin Has Neuroprotective Potential: Focus on Parkinson's Disease and Migraine. Front Neurol. 2017; 8: 333. https://www.ncbi.nlm.nih.gov/pmc/articles/PMC5517396/

287. Bhusal A, Banks SW. Riboflavin Deficiency. [Updated 2017 Nov 29]. In: StatPearls [Internet]. Treasure Island (FL): StatPearls Publishing; 2018 Jan-. https://www.ncbi.nlm.nih.gov/books/NBK470460/

288. TheOsimani, Berger, Friedman J, Katz BS-Porat, Abarbanel JM. Neuropsychology of vitamin B12 deficiency in elderly dementia patients and control subjects. J Geriatr Psychiatry Neurol. 2005; 18 (1): 33-8. https://www.ncbi.nlm.nih.gov/pubmed/15681626

289. Oudshoorn C, Mattace-raso FU, Van der velde N, Colin EM, Van der cammen TJ. Higher serum vitamin D3 levels are associated with better cognitive performance in patients with Alzheimer's disease. Dement Geriatr Cogn Disord. 2008; 25 (6): 539-43. https://www.ncbi.nlm.nih.gov/pubmed/18503256

290. Lin L, Huang QX, Yang SS, Chu J, Wang JZ, Tian Q. Melatonin in Alzheimer's Disease. International Journal of Molecular Sciences. 2013; 14 (7): 14575-14593. doi: 10.3390/ijms140714575. https://www.ncbi.nlm.nih.gov/pmc/articles/PMC3742260/

291. Watanabe F, Yabuta Y, Bito T, Teng F. Vitamin B12-Containing Plant Food Sources for Vegetarians. Nutrients. 2014; 6 (5): 1861-1873. doi: 10.3390/nu6051861. https://www.ncbi.nlm.nih.gov/pmc/articles/PMC4042564/

292. Kumudha A, Selvakumar S, Dilshad P, Vaidyanathan G, Thakur MS, Sarada R. Methylcobalamin - the form of vitamin B12 identified and characterized in Chlorella vulgaris. Food Chem. 2015; 170: 316-20. https://www.ncbi.nlm.nih.gov/pubmed/25306351

293. Article: http://www.netdoctor.co.uk/medicines/diet-and-nutrition/a6753/folic-acid-dosage-and-how-to-take/

294. Czeizel AE, Dudás I, Vereczkey A, Bánhidy F. Folate deficiency and folic acid supplementation: the prevention of neural-tube defects and congenital heart defects. Nutrients. 2013;5(11):4760-75.
https://www.ncbi.nlm.nih.gov/pubmed/24284617

295. Greenberg JA, Bell SJ, Guan Y, Yu Y. Folic Acid Supplementation and Pregnancy: More Than Just Neural Tube Defect Prevention. Reviews in Obstetrics and Gynecology. 2011;4(2):52-59.
https://www.ncbi.nlm.nih.gov/pmc/articles/PMC3218540/

296. Dhur A, Galan P, Hercberg S. Folate status and the immune system. Prog Food Nutr Sci. 1991;15(1-2):43-60.
https://www.ncbi.nlm.nih.gov/pubmed/1887065

297. Odewole OA, Williamson RS, Zakai NA, et al. Near-elimination of folate-deficiency anemia by mandatory folic acid fortification in older US adults: Reasons for Geographic and Racial Differences in Stroke study 2003-2007. Am J Clin Nutr. 2013;98(4):1042-7. https://www.ncbi.nlm.nih.gov/pubmed/23945721

298. Wierzbicki AS. Homocysteine and cardiovascular disease: a review of the evidence. Diab Vasc Dis Res. 2007;4(2):143-50.
https://www.ncbi.nlm.nih.gov/pubmed/17654449

299. Casas JP, Bautista LE, Smeeth L, Sharma P, Hingorani AD. Homocysteine and stroke: evidence on a causal link from mendelian randomisation. Lancet. 2005;365(9455):224-32. https://www.ncbi.nlm.nih.gov/pubmed/15652605

300. Li Y, Huang T, Zheng Y, Muka T, Troup J, Hu FB. Folic Acid Supplementation and the Risk of Cardiovascular Diseases: A Meta-Analysis of Randomized Controlled Trials. Journal of the American Heart Association: Cardiovascular and Cerebrovascular Disease. 2016;5(8):e003768. doi:10.1161/JAHA.116.003768. https://www.ncbi.nlm.nih.gov/pmc/articles/PMC5015297/

301. Reynolds EH. Folic acid, ageing, depression, and dementia. BMJ. 2002;324(7352):1512-5.
https://www.ncbi.nlm.nih.gov/pmc/articles/PMC1123448/

302. Tchantchou F, Shea TB. Folate deprivation, the methionine cycle, and Alzheimer's disease. Vitam Horm. 2008;79:83-97.
https://www.ncbi.nlm.nih.gov/pubmed/18804692

303. Choi SW, Mason JB. Folate status: effects on pathways of colorectal carcinogenesis. J Nutr. 2002;132(8 Suppl):2413S-2418S.
https://www.ncbi.nlm.nih.gov/pubmed/12163703

304. Blount BC, Mack MM, Wehr CM, et al. Folate deficiency causes uracil misincorporation into human DNA and chromosome breakage: implications for cancer and neuronal damage. Proc Natl Acad Sci USA. 1997;94(7):3290-5.
https://www.ncbi.nlm.nih.gov/pubmed/9096386

305. Patanwala I, King MJ, Barrett DA, et al. Folic acid handling by the human gut: implications for food fortification and supplementation. Am J Clin Nutr. 2014;100(2):593-9. https://www.ncbi.nlm.nih.gov/pubmed/24944062

306. Lamers Y, Prinz-langenohl R, Brämswig S, Pietrzik K. Red blood cell folate concentrations increase more after supplementation with [6S]-5-methyltetrahydrofolate than with folic acid in women of childbearing age. Am J Clin Nutr. 2006;84(1):156-61. https://www.ncbi.nlm.nih.gov/pubmed/16825690

307. Scaglione F, Panzavolta G. Folate, folic acid and 5-methyltetrahydrofolate are not the same thing. Xenobiotica. 2014;44(5):480-8 https://www.ncbi.nlm.nih.gov/pubmed/24494987

308. Article: https://lup.lub.lu.se/student-papers/search/publication/8894568

309. Vincent JB. Chromium: celebrating 50 years as an essential element?. Dalton Trans. 2010;39(16):3787-94. https://www.ncbi.nlm.nih.gov/pubmed/20372701

310. Vincent JB. Chromium: is it essential, pharmacologically relevant, or toxic?. Met Ions Life Sci. 2013;13:171-98.
https://www.ncbi.nlm.nih.gov/pubmed/24470092

311. Schachter S, Nelson RW, Kirk CA. Oral chromium picolinate and control of glycemia in insulin-treated diabetic dogs. J Vet Intern Med. 2001;15(4):379-84. https://www.ncbi.nlm.nih.gov/pubmed/11467597

312. Vincent JB. New Evidence against Chromium as an Essential Trace Element. J Nutr. 2017;147(12):2212-2219.
https://www.ncbi.nlm.nih.gov/pubmed/29021369

313. Ashoush S, Abou-gamrah A, Bayoumy H, Othman N. Chromium picolinate reduces insulin resistance in polycystic ovary syndrome: Randomized controlled trial. J Obstet Gynaecol Res. 2016;42(3):279-85.
https://www.ncbi.nlm.nih.gov/pubmed/26663540

314. Drake TC, Rudser KD, Seaquist ER, Saeed A. Chromium infusion in hospitalized patients with severe insulin resistance: a retrospective analysis. Endocr Pract. 2012;18(3):394-8.
https://www.ncbi.nlm.nih.gov/pubmed/22297054

315. Broadhurst CL, Domenico P. Clinical studies on chromium picolinate supplementation in diabetes mellitus—a review. Diabetes Technol Ther. 2006;8(6):677-87. https://www.ncbi.nlm.nih.gov/pubmed/17109600

316. Cerulli J, Grabe DW, Gauthier I, Malone M, Mcgoldrick MD. Chromium picolinate toxicity. Ann Pharmacother. 1998;32(4):428-31.
https://www.ncbi.nlm.nih.gov/pubmed/9562138

317. Yakubov E, Buchfelder M, Eyüpoglu IY, Savaskan NE. Selenium action in neuro-oncology. Biol Trace Elem Res. 2014;161(3):246-54.
https://www.ncbi.nlm.nih.gov/pubmed/25164034

318. Beck MA, Levander OA, Handy J. Selenium deficiency and viral infection. J Nutr. 2003;133(5 Suppl 1):1463S-7S.
https://www.ncbi.nlm.nih.gov/pubmed/12730444/

319. Dhur A, Galan P, Hercberg S. Relationship between selenium, immunity and resistance against infection. Comp Biochem Physiol C, Comp Pharmacol Toxicol. 1990;96(2):271-80. https://www.ncbi.nlm.nih.gov/pubmed/1980438

320. Rayman MP, Rayman MP. The argument for increasing selenium intake. Proc Nutr Soc. 2002;61(2):203-15. https://www.ncbi.nlm.nih.gov/pubmed/12133202

321. Kamwesiga J, Mutabazi V, Kayumba J, et al. Effect of selenium supplementation on CD4+ T-cell recovery, viral suppression and morbidity of HIV-infected patients in Rwanda: a randomized controlled trial. AIDS (London, England). 2015;29(9):1045-1052. doi:10.1097/QAD.0000000000000673. https://www.ncbi.nlm.nih.gov/pmc/articles/PMC4444428/

322. Campa A, Baum MK. Role of selenium in HIV/AIDS. In: Selenium: Its Molecular Biology and Role in Human Health, edited by Hatfield DL, Berry MJ, Gladyshev VN, editors. New York: Springer, 2012, p. 383–397

323. Kaushal N, Gandhi UH, Nelson SM, Narayan V, Prabhu KS.Selenium and inflamation. In: Selenium: Its Molecular Biology and Role in Human Health, edited by Hatfield DL, Berry MJ, Gladyshev VN, editors. New York: Springer, 2012, p. 443–456

324. Article: https://www.ncbi.nlm.nih.gov/pmc/articles/PMC4302047/

325. Handy DE, Loscalzo J. Selenoproteins in cardiovascular redox pathology. In: Selenium: Its Molecular Biology and Role in Human Health, edited by Hatfield DL, Berry MJ, Gladyshev VN, editors. New York: Springer, 2012, p. 249–259

326. Handy DE, Loscalzo J. Selenoproteins in cardiovascular redox pathology. In: Selenium: Its Molecular Biology and Role in Human Health, edited by Hatfield DL, Berry MJ, Gladyshev VN, editors. New York: Springer, 2012, p. 249–259

327. Jackson MI, Combs GF. Selenium as a cancer preventive agent. In: Selenium: Its Molecular Biology and Role in Human Health, edited by Hatfield DL, Berry MJ, Gladyshev VN, editors. New York: Springer, 2012, p. 313–323

328. Berggren M, Sittadjody S, Song Z, Samira JL, Burd R, Meuillet EJ. Sodium Selenite Increases the Activity of the Tumor Suppressor Protein, PTEN in DU-145 Prostate Cancer Cells. Nutrition and cancer. 2009;61(3):322-331. doi:10.1080/01635580802521338. https://www.ncbi.nlm.nih.gov/pmc/articles/PMC4049328/

329. Turanov AA, Malinouski M, Gladyshev VN. Selenium and male reproduction. In: Selenium: Its Molecular Biology and Role in Human Health, edited by Hatfield DL, Berry MJ, Gladyshev VN, editors. New York: Springer, 2012, p. 409–417

330. Berggren M, Sittadjody S, Song Z, Samira JL, Burd R, Meuillet EJ. Sodium Selenite Increases the Activity of the Tumor Suppressor Protein, PTEN in DU-145 Prostate Cancer Cells. Nutrition and cancer. 2009;61(3):322-331. doi:10.1080/01635580802521338. https://www.ncbi.nlm.nih.gov/pubmed/11215512/

331. Van zuuren EJ, Albusta AY, Fedorowicz Z, Carter B, Pijl H. Selenium supplementation for Hashimoto's thyroiditis. Cochrane Database Syst Rev. 2013;(6):CD010223. https://www.ncbi.nlm.nih.gov/pubmed/23744563

332. Duntas LH. The Role of Iodine and Selenium in Autoimmune Thyroiditis. Horm Metab Res. 2015;47(10):721-6. https://www.ncbi.nlm.nih.gov/pubmed/26361258

333. Dharmasena A. Selenium supplementation in thyroid associated ophthalmopathy: an update. International Journal of Ophthalmology.

2014;7(2):365-375. doi:10.3980/j.issn.2222-3959.2014.02.31.
https://www.ncbi.nlm.nih.gov/pmc/articles/PMC4003098/

334. See KA, Lavercombe PS, Dillon J, Ginsberg R. Accidental death from acute selenium poisoning. Med J Aust. 2006;185(7):388-9.
https://www.ncbi.nlm.nih.gov/pubmed/17014408

335. Xu JW, Shi XM, Yin ZX, Liu YZ, Zhai Y, Zeng Y. [Investigation and analysis of plasma trace elements of oldest elderly in longevity areas in China]. Zhonghua Yu Fang Yi Xue Za Zhi. 2010;44(2):119-22.
https://www.ncbi.nlm.nih.gov/pubmed/20388331

336. Akbaraly NT, Arnaud J, Hininger-favier I, Gourlet V, Roussel AM, Berr C. Selenium and mortality in the elderly: results from the EVA study. Clin Chem. 2005;51(11):2117-23. https://www.ncbi.nlm.nih.gov/pubmed/16123147

337. Article: http://www.lifeextension.com/magazine/2015/11/how-to-obtain-optimal-benefits-from-selenium/page-01

338. Suhajda A, Hegóczki J, Janzsó B, Pais I, Vereczkey G. Preparation of selenium yeasts I. Preparation of selenium-enriched Saccharomyces cerevisiae. J Trace Elem Med Biol. 2000;14(1):43-7.
https://www.ncbi.nlm.nih.gov/pubmed/10836533

339. Rayman MP. The use of high-selenium yeast to raise selenium status: how does it measure up?. Br J Nutr. 2004;92(4):557-73.
https://www.ncbi.nlm.nih.gov/pubmed/15522125

340. Ip C, Lisk DJ. Bioactivity of selenium from Brazil nut for cancer prevention and selenoenzyme maintenance. Nutr Cancer. 1994;21(3):203-12.
https://www.ncbi.nlm.nih.gov/pubmed/8072875

341. Silva junior EC, Wadt LHO, Silva KE, et al. Natural variation of selenium in Brazil nuts and soils from the Amazon region. Chemosphere. 2017;188:650-658.
https://www.ncbi.nlm.nih.gov/pubmed/28923728

342. Colpo E, Vilanova CD de A, Brenner Reetz LG, et al. A Single Consumption of High Amounts of the Brazil Nuts Improves Lipid Profile of Healthy Volunteers. *Journal of Nutrition and Metabolism*. 2013;2013:653185.
doi:10.1155/2013/653185.
https://www.ncbi.nlm.nih.gov/pmc/articles/PMC3693158/

343. Evans M, Rumberger JA, Azumano I, Napolitano JJ, Citrolo D, Kamiya T. Pantethine, a derivative of vitamin B5, favorably alters total, LDL and non-HDL cholesterol in low to moderate cardiovascular risk subjects eligible for statin therapy: a triple-blinded placebo and diet-controlled investigation. *Vascular Health and Risk Management*. 2014;10:89-100. doi:10.2147/VHRM.S57116.
https://www.ncbi.nlm.nih.gov/pmc/articles/PMC3942300/

344. Article: https://www.consumerlab.com/answers/does-coq10-have-to-be-taken-with-food/water_soluble_CoQ10/

345. Oleck S, Ventura HO. Coenzyme Q10 and Utility in Heart Failure: Just Another Supplement?. Curr Heart Fail Rep. 2016;13(4):190-5.
https://www.ncbi.nlm.nih.gov/pubmed/27333901

346. Jankowski J, Korzeniowska K, Cieślewicz A, Jabłecka A. Coenzyme Q10 — A new player in the treatment of heart failure?. Pharmacol Rep. 2016;68(5):1015-9. https://www.ncbi.nlm.nih.gov/pubmed/27428763

347. Hargreaves IP. Coenzyme Q10 as a therapy for mitochondrial disease. Int J Biochem Cell Biol. 2014;49:105-11. https://www.ncbi.nlm.nih.gov/pubmed/24495877

348. Ott M, Gogvadze V, Orrenius S, Zhivotovsky B. Mitochondria, oxidative stress and cell death. Apoptosis. 2007;12(5):913-22. https://www.ncbi.nlm.nih.gov/pubmed/17453160

349. Littarru GP, Tiano L. Bioenergetic and antioxidant properties of coenzyme Q10: recent developments. Mol Biotechnol. 2007;37(1):31-7 https://www.ncbi.nlm.nih.gov/pubmed/17914161

350. Dhanasekaran M, Ren J. The emerging role of coenzyme Q-10 in aging, neurodegeneration, cardiovascular disease, cancer and diabetes mellitus. Curr Neurovasc Res. 2005;2(5):447-59. https://www.ncbi.nlm.nih.gov/pubmed/16375724

351. Mortensen SA, Vadhanavikit S, Baandrup U, Folkers K. Long-term coenzyme Q10 therapy: a major advance in the management of resistant myocardial failure. Drugs Exp Clin Res. 1985;11(8):581-93. https://www.ncbi.nlm.nih.gov/pubmed/3836876

352. Fotino AD, Thompson-paul AM, Bazzano LA. Effect of coenzyme Q_{10} supplementation on heart failure: a meta-analysis. Am J Clin Nutr. 2013;97(2):268-75. https://www.ncbi.nlm.nih.gov/pubmed/23221577

353. Berman M, Erman A, Ben-gal T, et al. Coenzyme Q10 in patients with end-stage heart failure awaiting cardiac transplantation: a randomized, placebo-controlled study. Clin Cardiol. 2004;27(5):295-9. https://www.ncbi.nlm.nih.gov/pubmed/15188947

354. Langsjoen H, Langsjoen P, Langsjoen P, Willis R, Folkers K. Usefulness of coenzyme Q10 in clinical cardiology: a long-term study. Mol Aspects Med. 1994;15 Suppl:s165-75. https://www.ncbi.nlm.nih.gov/pubmed/7752828

355. Morisco C, Trimarco B, Condorelli M. Effect of coenzyme Q10 therapy in patients with congestive heart failure: a long-term multicenter randomized study. Clin Investig. 1993;71(8 Suppl):S134-6. https://www.ncbi.nlm.nih.gov/pubmed/8241697

356. Pepe S, Marasco SF, Haas SJ, Sheeran FL, Krum H, Rosenfeldt FL. Coenzyme Q10 in cardiovascular disease. Mitochondrion. 2007;7 Suppl:S154-67. https://www.ncbi.nlm.nih.gov/pubmed/17485243

357. Molyneux SL, Florkowski CM, Richards AM, Lever M, Young JM, George PM. Coenzyme Q10; an adjunctive therapy for congestive heart failure?. NZ Med J. 2009;122(1305):74-9. https://www.ncbi.nlm.nih.gov/pubmed/19966871

358. Somers-edgar TJ, Rosengren RJ. Coenzyme Q0 induces apoptosis and modulates the cell cycle in estrogen receptor negative breast cancer cells. Anticancer Drugs. 2009;20(1):33-40. https://www.ncbi.nlm.nih.gov/pubmed/18830129

359. Sandhir R, Sethi N, Aggarwal A, Khera A. Coenzyme Q10 treatment ameliorates cognitive deficits by modulating mitochondrial functions in surgically induced menopause. Neurochem Int. 2014;74:16-23. https://www.ncbi.nlm.nih.gov/pubmed/24780430

360. Duberley KE, Heales SJ, Abramov AY, et al. Effect of Coenzyme Q10 supplementation on mitochondrial electron transport chain activity and mitochondrial oxidative stress in Coenzyme Q10 deficient human neuronal cells. Int J Biochem Cell Biol. 2014;50:60-3. https://www.ncbi.nlm.nih.gov/pubmed/24534273

361. Somayajulu M, Mccarthy S, Hung M, Sikorska M, Borowy-borowski H, Pandey S. Role of mitochondria in neuronal cell death induced by oxidative stress; neuroprotection by Coenzyme Q10. Neurobiol Dis. 2005;18(3):618-27. https://www.ncbi.nlm.nih.gov/pubmed/15755687

362. Barca E, Kleiner G, Tang G, et al. Decreased Coenzyme Q10 Levels in Multiple System Atrophy Cerebellum. J Neuropathol Exp Neurol. 2016;75(7):663-72. https://www.ncbi.nlm.nih.gov/pubmed/27235405

363. Schottlaender LV, Bettencourt C, Kiely AP, et al. Coenzyme Q10 Levels Are Decreased in the Cerebellum of Multiple-System Atrophy Patients. PLoS ONE. 2016;11(2):e0149557. https://www.ncbi.nlm.nih.gov/pubmed/26894433

364. Lee D, Kim KY, Shim MS, et al. Coenzyme Q10 ameliorates oxidative stress and prevents mitochondrial alteration in ischemic retinal injury. Apoptosis. 2014;19(4):603-14. https://www.ncbi.nlm.nih.gov/pubmed/24337820

365. Noh YH, Kim KY, Shim MS, et al. Inhibition of oxidative stress by coenzyme Q10 increases mitochondrial mass and improves bioenergetic function in optic nerve head astrocytes. Cell Death Dis. 2013;4:e820. https://www.ncbi.nlm.nih.gov/pubmed/24091663

366. Mezawa M, Takemoto M, Onishi S, et al. The reduced form of coenzyme Q10 improves glycemic control in patients with type 2 diabetes: an open label pilot study. Biofactors. 2012;38(6):416-21. https://www.ncbi.nlm.nih.gov/pubmed/22887051

367. Hodgson JM, Watts GF, Playford DA, Burke V, Croft KD. Coenzyme Q10 improves blood pressure and glycaemic control: a controlled trial in subjects with type 2 diabetes. Eur J Clin Nutr. 2002;56(11):1137-42. https://www.ncbi.nlm.nih.gov/pubmed/12428181

368. Ishikawa A, Homma Y. Beneficial effect of ubiquinol, the reduced form of coenzyme Q10, on cyclosporine nephrotoxicity. Int Braz J Urol. 2012;38(2):230-4. https://www.ncbi.nlm.nih.gov/pubmed/22555041

369. Hosoe K, Kitano M, Kishida H, Kubo H, Fujii K, Kitahara M. Study on safety and bioavailability of ubiquinol (Kaneka QH) after single and 4-week multiple oral administration to healthy volunteers. Regul Toxicol Pharmacol. 2007;47(1):19-28. https://www.ncbi.nlm.nih.gov/pubmed/16919858

370. Langsjoen PH, Langsjoen AM. Comparison study of plasma coenzyme Q10 levels in healthy subjects supplemented with ubiquinol versus ubiquinone. Clin

Pharmacol Drug Dev. 2014;3(1):13-7.
https://www.ncbi.nlm.nih.gov/pubmed/27128225
371. Failla ML, Chitchumroonchokchai C, Aoki F. Increased bioavailability of ubiquinol compared to that of ubiquinone is due to more efficient micellarization during digestion and greater GSH-dependent uptake and basolateral secretion by Caco-2 cells. J Agric Food Chem. 2014;62(29):7174-82.
https://www.ncbi.nlm.nih.gov/pubmed/24979483
372. Crescenti A, Puiggròs F, Colomé A, et al. [Anti-allergy effect of a plant mixture of Herniaria glabra, Agropyron repens, Equisetum arvense and Sambucus nigra (Herbensurina®) in the prevention of experimentally induced nephrolithiasis in rats]. Arch Esp Urol. 2015; 68 (10): 739-49.
https://www.ncbi.nlm.nih.gov/pubmed/26634575
373. Ghane shahrbaf F, Assadi F. Drug-induced renal disorders. J Renal Inj Prev. 2015; 4 (3): 57-60. https://www.ncbi.nlm.nih.gov/pmc/articles/PMC4594214/
374. Gøtzsche PC. Our prescription drugs kill us in large numbers. Pol Arch Med Wewn. 2014; 124 (11): 628-34.
https://www.ncbi.nlm.nih.gov/pubmed/25355584